Basic Surgical Skills Manual

Basic Surgical Skills Manual

Iain Skinner

The McGraw-Hill Companies, Inc.

Sydney New York San Francisco Auckland
Bangkok Bogotá Caracas Hong Kong
Kuala Lumpur Lisbon London Madrid
Mexico City Milan New Delhi San Juan
Seoul Singapore Taipei Toronto

McGraw·Hill Australia
*A Division of The **McGraw·Hill** Companies*

NOTICE
Medicine is an ever-changing science. As new research and clinical experience broaden our knowledge, changes in treatment and drug therapy are required. The editors and the publisher of this work have checked with sources believed to be reliable in their efforts to provide information that is complete and generally in accord with the standards accepted at the time of publication. However, in view of the possibility of human error or changes in medical sciences, neither the editors, nor the publisher, nor any other party who has been involved in the preparation or publication of this work warrants that the information contained herein is in every respect accurate or complete. Readers are encouraged to confirm the information contained herein with other sources. For example, and in particular, readers are advised to check the product information sheet included in the package of each drug they plan to administer to be certain that the information contained in this book is accurate and that changes have not been made in the recommended dose or in the contraindications for administration. This recommendation is of particular importance in connection with new or infrequently used drugs.

Text © 2000 Iain Skinner
Illustrations and design © 2000 McGraw-Hill Book Company Australia Pty Limited
Additional owners of copyright material are acknowledged in on-page credits.

DEXON, DEXON II, MAXON SURGILENE, NOVAFIL and SOFTGUT are trademarks of Davis and Geck. DYLOC, VILENE are trademarks of Dynek Sutures Pty Ltd. PROLENE, MONOCRYL, VICRYL, PDS and PDS II are all trademarks of Ethicon Inc.

Apart from any fair dealing for the purposes of study, research, criticism or review, as permitted under the Copyright Act, no part may be reproduced by any process without written permission. Enquiries should be made to the publisher, marked for the attention of the Permissions Editor, at the address below.

Every effort has been made to trace and acknowledge copyright material. Should any infringement have occurred accidentally the authors and publishers tender their apologies.

Copying for educational purposes
Under the copying provisions of the *Copyright Act*, copies of parts of this book may be made by an educational institution. An agreement exists between the Copyright Agency Limited (CAL) and the relevant educational authority (Department of Education, university, TAFE, etc.) to pay a licence fee for such copying. It is not necessary to keep records of copying except where the relevant educational authority has undertaken to do so by arrangement with the Copyright Agency Limited.

For further information on the CAL licence agreements with educational institutions, contact the Copyright Agency Limited, Level 19, 157 Liverpool Street, Sydney NSW 2000. Where no such agreement exists, the copyright owner is entitled to claim payment in respect of any copies made.

Enquiries concerning copyright in McGraw-Hill publications should be directed to the Permissions Editor at the address below.

National Library of Australia Cataloguing-in-Publication data:

Skinner, Iain.
Basic surgical skills manual.

Bibliography.
Includes index.
ISBN 0 074 70608 X.

1. Surgery, Operative—Handbooks, manuals, etc. 2. Surgical instruments and apparatus—Handbooks, manuals, etc. 3. Wounds and injuries—Surgery—Handbooks, manuals, etc. 4. Anesthesiology—Handbooks, manuals, etc. I. Title.

617.9

Published in Australia by
McGraw-Hill Book Company Australia Pty Limited
4 Barcoo Street, Roseville NSW 2069, Australia
Acquisitions Editors: Kristen Baragwanath, Meiling Voon
Production Editor: Megan Lowe
Editor: Jo Rudd
Designer: Kimberly Taliai, blue orange
Illustrator: Lorenzo Lucia, Tech View Studio
Typeset in Gill Sans Light by Midland Typesetters
Printed on 80 gsm woodfree by Prowell Productions, Hong Kong

Foreword

The nature of basic skills training in surgery has changed dramatically in recent years. For centuries, the development of operative skills has depended on apprenticeship, where the acknowledged masters of the craft have demonstrated to their juniors the niceties of surgical technique with varying levels of ability and educational skill. Much has depended on the innate ability of both master and pupil and skill development has not always been supervised as closely as it should be—the best surgeons are not always the best or most capable assistants. This apprenticeship system has depended on the willingness (or perhaps the ignorance) of patients to accept that surgical procedures will often be conducted on them by apprentices of varying levels of skill and experience, a situation which is changing rapidly.

As an understanding of the proper processes of education and acquisition of skills has developed, and with changing patient expectations and the financial constraints of modern health care, it has become apparent that there must be more effective, more consistent and more appropriate methods for the acquisition, testing and maintenance of surgical skills.

The different surgical specialties have varied in their appreciation of these issues, with the ophthalmologists and the orthopaedic surgeons leading the way in the provision of courses to develop technical skill with the use of tissues and/or simulators rather than patients. These general principles have now been accepted by surgery in general, and the Royal Colleges in the United Kingdom, and more recently in Australasia, have developed courses for both surgeons in training and practising surgeons, who can acquire and be certified in new techniques as they are developed in a rapidly changing world.

Iain Skinner has participated in these developments both as a pupil and a teacher in the United Kingdom and in Australia. Thus he is well placed to have authored this text, which brings together several areas of basic surgical principles, instrumentation, materials and techniques which are essential areas of knowledge and skill for surgical trainees as they pass through basic to advanced training. The apprenticeship system will persist, since it maintains many virtues in spite of its deficiencies. However, it must be complemented by texts such as this if trainees are to reach their full potential.

GORDON J.A. CLUNIE
Chairman, Court of Examiners, Royal Australasian College of Surgeons
Emeritus Professor of Surgery, University of Melbourne.

About the author

Iain James Skinner

Iain James Skinner was educated at Melbourne Church of England Grammar School and the University of Melbourne, graduating MBBS in 1988. After initial residency posts at the Royal Melbourne Hospital he spent a year each at the University of Melbourne Anatomy School and the Royal Devon and Exeter Hospital in the UK, returning to Australia in 1993. Iain entered Advanced Surgical Training with the Royal Australasian College of Surgeons in 1994 and was awarded Fellowship of the Royal Australasian College of Surgeons in 1999.

Iain's practical and research interests in Surgical Skills Education began while in England. He has been actively involved in practical skills course development at the Royal Melbourne Hospital, Western Hospital (Melbourne) and the Royal Australasian College of Surgeons. His current research project, looking at predictors of surgical skill, is under preparation as the thesis for a Master of Surgery (Research) degree. This manual came about as a direct result of the need for a basic skill textbook in this project.

Iain is married to Geraldine and has two children, Alexander and Olivia. At present he is on a surgical attachment in the United Kingdom and plans to return to general surgical practice in Melbourne sometime in the next millennium.

Contents

Foreword	v
About the author	vi
Introduction	xi

1 The basic principles of wound management   1
Assessment of wounds	1
The pathology of wound healing	24
The surgical management of wounds	32
Conclusions	39
Further reading	39

2 Surgical instruments and their uses   40
Cutting instruments	41
Grasping instruments	53
Retracting instruments	74
Other instruments	83
Surgical diathermy	86
Further reading	90

3 Suture materials and surgical needles   91
Surgical needles	92
Suture sizes	97
Suture materials	98
Further reading	111

4 Basic surgical skills — 112

Basic principles and the operative field — 112
Basic suturing techniques — 116
Surgical knot tying — 130
Basic surgical techniques — 144
Basic assisting techniques — 163
Further reading — 170

5 Local anaesthetics and their uses — 171

Introduction — 171
Local anaesthetics and dosages — 176
Local anaesthetic toxicity — 178
Administration methods — 181
Local infiltration anaesthesia — 184
Further reading — 186

6 Sterile technique — 187

Introduction — 187
The principles and practice of sterile technique — 188
Conclusions — 207
Further reading — 207

7 Safety in the operating theatre — 210

The surgeon and scrub team — 210
The patient — 214
Other personnel — 218

Glossary — 220
Index — 229

Acknowledgments

My thanks must go to the following people: Professor Gordon Clunie who inspired my interest in surgery, supported me in the early years of my training and encouraged my interest in surgical education; Mr Peter Gregory; Dr Andrew Robertson; Ms Jan Stevens; Ms Jan Jackson; Pierre and Janna and Lindsay from the University of Melbourne Department of Surgery; Julianne and Amanda of Melbourne Private Hospital theatres; Lucy and Lily and Helen (formerly) of Royal Melbourne Hospital theatres; Dr Rob Moulds and Dr Christine Penfold of the Royal Melbourne Hospital Clinical School; and Dorothy and Betty (both formerly) of the RMH Clinical School, all of whom had direct and indirect input into the production of this book; all the surgeons, and other doctors, with whom I have worked for teaching me the skills and setting the example for me to follow; my parents, Catherine and James Skinner, for believing in my dream and helping me to realise it; and last, but most importantly, my wife Geraldine, my son Alexander and my daughter Olivia, for accepting me and my commitment to surgery. To these last five people goes all my love.

Introduction

> We need a system, and we shall surely have it, which will produce not only surgeons but surgeons of the highest type, men [sic] who will stimulate the first youths of our country to study surgery and to devote their energies and their lives to raising the standard of surgical science.
>
> William Halsted, 'The Training of the Surgeon', Yale Lecture 1904

The training of a surgeon

Skill acquisition in surgery has traditionally followed an apprenticeship model. The more experienced practitioners (surgeons) demonstrate their preferred technique to the apprentice (registrar) and this is repeated under levels of decreasing supervision until competence to perform the task solo is attained. The end-point of this training process must also include the considered, careful, gentle, accurate and safe manipulation of tissues for the appropriate reasons. History has demonstrated validity in this method, as we continue to produce surgeons of excellence, but there is always potential for restrictions in operative experience, instruction in poor techniques, development and perpetuation of bad habits and minimally experienced personnel being used to teach basic skills to novices.

Is this system adequate, then, if the basics of practice are poorly taught, or even not taught, and need to be acquired by osmosis from watching? Is it also warranted to use patients as the 'material' upon which these early skills are practised? Intuitively we would think not, but to change this precedent we must look to the alternatives and choose a proven better option.

What alternatives do we have to 'live training'? If we look at sportspeople and musicians, they are usually involved in complex training drills and simulated performances prior to the main event. Similarly, pilots spend many hours in mechanical flight simulators rehearsing routine and emergency scenarios before taking on the responsibility of a plane full of people. Studies of expert skill acquisition have shown clear patterns. Three factors seem related to superior skills—an 'innate ability' to develop the skills, early age of initial skills training and regular, intensive goal-directed practice. All these elements appear to be lacking in surgical training. There are, as yet, no tests or objective measures of potential skills ability. Training is usually commenced at postgraduate level, often when trainees are older than 25 years, and skills practice is sporadic, patient-based and not directed to specific goals. To combat these inadequacies we should be looking at predictors and simulators for both the initial instruction and the subsequent development of surgical skills.

Happily, some evidence exists that simulations in surgical training do work. Individual proficiency in microvascular techniques, vascular anastomoses and other procedural skills has been shown to improve with the use of training models. These models range from synthetic material mimicking the real, through preserved and fresh animal viscera to live anaesthetised animals. Now virtual reality simulators are being developed in which full-screen goggles and pressure pad gloves will deliver the sight and feel of a normal human procedure by computer generation.

In looking at the rationale for teaching skills through simulators we must also take into account the opportunities for 'live training'. Unfortunately, our health-care system has developed a significant fiscal consciousness. Turnover must increase, turnover times decrease and we must all do more with less to keep standards the same. The same is true for training. Reductions in bed numbers, the need for a more rapid turnover and the strict training requirements for Surgical Registrars have all conspired to restrict the theatre time available for the teaching of basic skills to residents and students. The once, almost traditional, 'intern's appendix' is a rarity, and students, if they do get to scrub, are used mostly to hold retractors in long complex procedures where they can see little and understand even less.

As leaders in the training of surgeons, the Royal College of Surgeons in both England and Scotland are presently engaged in running basic and masterclass workshops in all aspects of operative surgery. Dedicated skills-training facilities have been built specifically to house these courses. Faculties of surgeon-educators have been seconded to develop, run and assess the various levels of skills-training workshops. It is now a requirement of training that all candidates for higher surgical examinations must have completed prescribed workshops in both basic and advanced surgical skills before being allowed to sit.

The Royal Australasian College of Surgeons (RACS) has been quick to follow this lead and is presently developing a new system of basic and advanced surgical training which will incorporate a skills component. It is hoped that this manual will aid the training process by providing an early introduction, for all doctors, to the skills required by a surgeon.

Specific aims of this manual

This basic surgical skills manual has been written to provide an introduction to the development, and appropriate use, of a variety of essential surgical skills. The manual assumes minimal knowledge of the subject and contains the basic information required by medical students, junior surgical trainees, procedural general practitioners, emergency department physicians and theatre staff to develop an understanding of surgical skills.

It should be self-evident that learning the motor element of these skills is only one part of training a surgeon. An understanding of the situations in which the skills should be used (the *when*) and the principles behind those skills (the *why*) is the real basis of surgical practice, without which the ability to perform the task (the *how*) is useless.

In writing a manual such as this it is inevitable that a subjective element will be present. The lessons I have learnt from my teachers, and the hospitals where I have worked, will surface. What I aim to present is a skeleton on which you may build your surgical abilities. '*Safe, simple, sensible and humble*' should be the mantra of the surgeon and I believe the lessons to be learnt from this book follow these principles.

What this book does not contain is all the skills you will need as a surgeon. These still need to be developed as apprentice to a master over a significant period of time. Listen to everyone who will teach you, take nothing for granted or at face value and learn to cultivate the best points of practice you see demonstrated. But, above all, use all your skills, all your mind and all of your heart to care for those people who will inevitably seek your help in the years to come.

Iain J. Skinner
Kent UK 1999

The basic principles of wound management

The initial assessment and subsequent management of wounds is a cornerstone of surgical practice, whether under the strict aseptic conditions of theatre or in the minor procedure rooms of emergency departments and general practice surgeries. The manual skills and decision making involved in the management phase are inevitably guided by an appropriate assessment of the wound. To make this thorough assessment an understanding of the mechanisms by which wounds are caused, and the ramifications of these different types of wound is needed. Finally, an understanding of wound healing and the factors affecting this complete the basic skills required for excellence in wound care.

Assessment of wounds

Assessment of wound type

The decision-making process in wound management must begin with assessment of the wound itself and consideration of the ramifications of how the wound was made. By necessity, the site of a wound and the amount of tissue loss will also impact on the management but details of this are left to more specialised texts (see Further Reading). Once fully assessed, management decisions can be made to maximise the wound's chance of uncomplicated healing.

One schema by which wounds may be classified is shown in Table 1.1 (pp. 4–5). This provides four classes of wound and relates to a combination of situation, mechanism, contamination and likelihood of infection. The lower a wound is rated (out of 4) the more likely that primary closure will be possible. Reclassification of a wound is possible by either complete excision in a sterile environment, thereby converting any wound to a type 1, or by extensive debridement and copious irrigation with conversion to a type 2 at best.

Type 1 wounds are essentially those made in an operating theatre or other sterile environment where no contaminated tissues are breached. These include procedure on the body walls and all non-contaminated deep tissues (e.g. thyroid gland, blood vessels, brain and bones). They suffer minimal contamination by airborne particles and heal with a negligible risk of infection. Primary wound closure (see later) is the method of choice. Any other type of wound may be converted to a type 1 by complete excision of the original wound in all planes.

Type 2 wounds are those clean and tidy incisional wounds inflicted by a sharp cutting implement in a non-sterile environment, or those wounds in operative procedures where a non-infected tract (e.g. small bowel or bronchial tree) has been opened with minimal macroscopic contamination. The risk of wound infection is still low and these wounds should be primarily closed after some form of wound toilet. Type 3 and 4 wounds can effectively be converted to a type 2 by wide debridement and copious wound irrigation.

Type 3 wounds are those untidy and contaminated wounds created in a dirty environment, wounds in operative procedures where an infected tract (e.g. infected bronchial tree or infected urological tract) or a dirty tract (e.g. large bowel or rectum) is opened, or wounds in procedures where gross and widespread contamination from a non-infected tract occurs. These wounds may require wide debridement and copious irrigation (i.e. conversion to a type 1 or 2 wound) before delayed primary or even primary closure. They have a significant risk of wound infection.

Type 4 wounds are infected, contaminated or devitalised wounds, open wounds of a duration greater than 12 hours, or operative wounds in areas of gross septic or faecal contamination. By definition they must not be closed unless confidently converted to a type 1 or 2 wound. Infection rates are high and the risk of gas gangrene or other necrotising infections exists.

Basic Surgical Skills

Type 1 wounds are surgically created in a sterile environment

(a) Type 1—clean wound

Type 2 wounds are created with a sharp instrument, are cleanly incised and minimally contaminated.

clean incision

(b) Type 2—clean contaminated wound

- torn clothing
- pieces of clothing and other foreign bodies
- torn deep fascia
- damaged muscle
- skin surface

Type 3 wounds are created with tearing or incision and are contaminated. There is no frank infection and minimal dead tissue. Type 3 wounds may become Type 4, over several hours, if left untreated.

(c) Type 3—contaminated wound

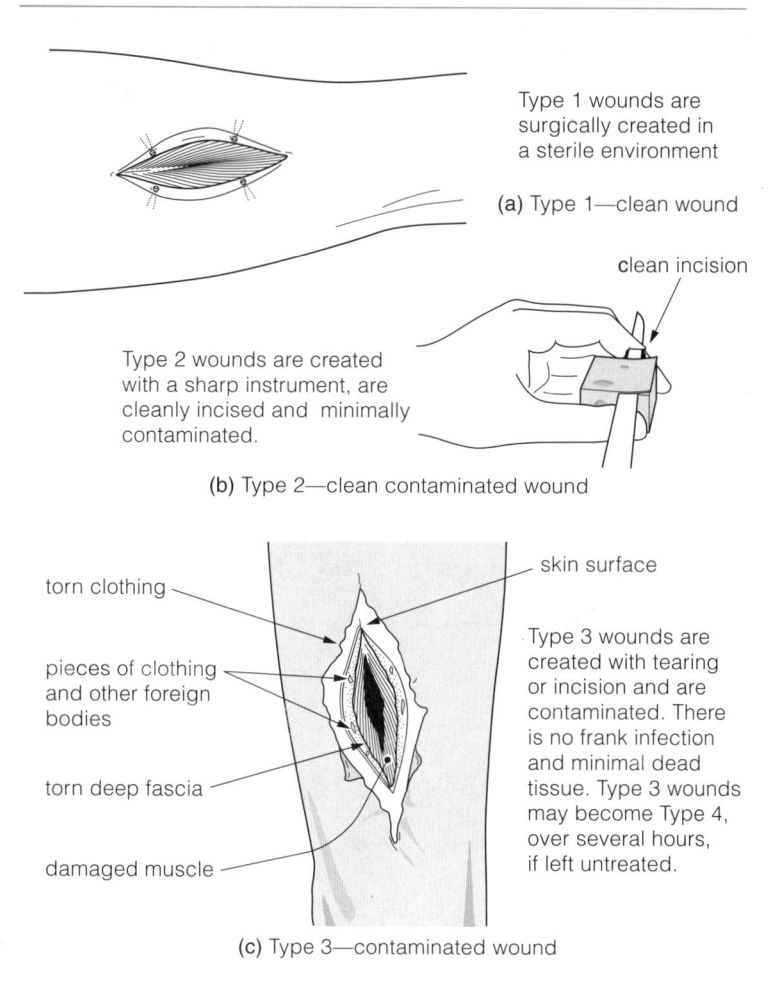

Type 4 wounds have severely damaged tissues with devascularisation and (often) gross contamination. Infection also constitutes part of this classification and may be superadded or the primary problem.

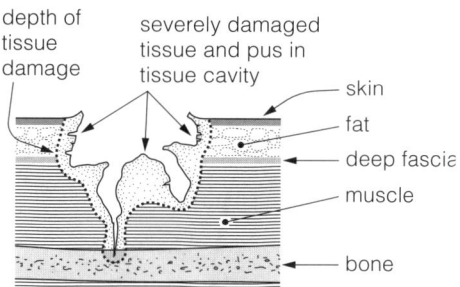

- depth of tissue damage
- severely damaged tissue and pus in tissue cavity
- skin
- fat
- deep fascia
- muscle
- bone

(d) Type 4—infected wound/grossly contaminated wound

Fig. 1.1 *Wound types*

The basic principles of wound management

The basic principles of wound management

Table 1.1 The four-tiered system of wound classification

Classification	Cause	Comments
1. Clean	• elective surgical wounds e.g. hernia surgery or breast biopsy	Low wound infection rate approximately <2% Routine primary closure
2. Contaminated—tidy	• low-velocity traumatic incisions • clean and sharp with local damage • contamination minor and brief • minor intraoperative contamination e.g.—kitchen knife/clean glass cut —small bowel or bronchial tree opened intraoperatively	Wound infection rate 1–5% Routine primary closure after some debridement and irrigation
3. Contaminated—untidy	• low velocity lacerating, tearing or bursting wounds • ragged and contused with gross local damage • contamination apparent and prolonged • major intraoperative contamination • all high-velocity injuries e.g.—crush injuries —garden tool injuries —bullet wounds —large bowel, infected bronchial tree or infected urinary tract opened intraoperatively	Wound infection rate 5–25% May be closed after wide debridement and copious irrigation or may require delayed primary closure

The basic principles of wound management

4. Dirty/Infected
- wounds with signs of infection such as erythema, cellulitis or pus
- grossly contaminated wounds
- more than 12 hours after injury
- severe tissue damage and excessive ischaemic tissue

e.g. – severe crush injuries
- penetrating abdominal trauma with hollow visceral perforation
- 'war wounds'
- cloth, shrapnel, faeces etc. in wound

Wound infection rate near to 50% if the wound is closed. May be closeable after total excision or wide debridement and copious irrigation but often requires healing by delayed primary closure or secondary intention

Assessment of wound mechanism

Mechanism of injury impacts greatly on the decisions made during wound management and information regarding this must be sought specifically on history. If details cannot be obtained, the appearance of a wound will often provide clues to its cause. Blunt or penetrating trauma, thermal injury, chemical injury, electrical injury and injury by ionising radiation are the six major mechanisms of injury. For completeness all six are dealt with here but, in reality, the most commonly treated wounds are caused by blunt trauma, penetrating trauma or heat. An appreciation of their effects and ramifications is essential for good wound management practices.

Table 1.2 summarises the mechanisms of wound causation.

Kinetic energy injury—closed (blunt)

This is a very common form of injury and results from either an object striking a person or a person striking an object. The essential component of this injury mechanism is deceleration with a subsequent transfer of kinetic energy. The two variants, however, have significantly different ramifications.

In the case of an object striking a person the major injury is usually localised to the region of impact. If we take the example of a cricket ball being hit into the head of a close fielder this becomes clearer. As the ball first strikes the skin of the forehead the tissue is compressed and may burst open as a stellate laceration. Blood vessels and underlying tissue also burst with subsequent haemorrhage and contusion (Fig. 1.2).

The energy transfer may then continue through the tissues resulting in deformation or fracturing of the underlying bone. Continuation of this force, combined with the bony deformation or fracture, may cause disruption of underlying brain tissues and meninges. Bleeding, contusion and possibly soft tissue fracture are common sequelae. Spikes of bone from a fracture may even penetrate the underlying tissue, causing similar injuries (Fig. 1.3). Finally, the forced compression of the brain against the back of the cranial vault, and its subsequent recoil, may result in damage to the frontal lobes (contre-coup injury) (Fig. 1.4).

When a person strikes an object, (e.g. the ground after a fall from a roof), there are several mechanisms of injury. The first is the direct strike of body parts causing localised blunt injuries, as above, at one or multiple sites. Equally important is the effect of deceleration on the

Basic Surgical Skills

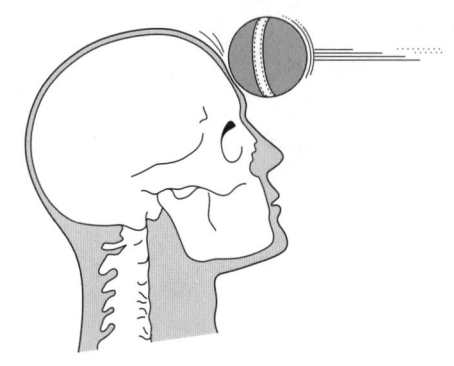

(a) Cricket ball strikes forehead compressing the skin and subcutaneous tissues and causing them to burst.

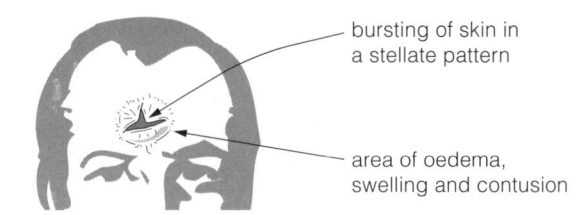

— bursting of skin in a stellate pattern

— area of oedema, swelling and contusion

(b) The burst laceration is usually stellate and raised due to both oedema and haematoma/contusion.

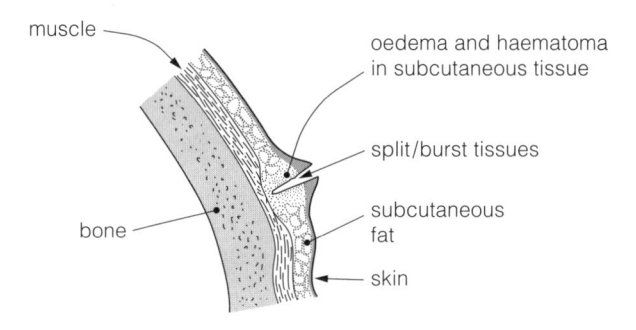

muscle

oedema and haematoma in subcutaneous tissue

split/burst tissues

subcutaneous fat

bone

skin

(c) Cross-section of burst/lacerated tissues showing oedema and haematoma.

Fig. 1.2 *Surface contact injury with transfer of kinetic energy*

Basic Surgical Skills

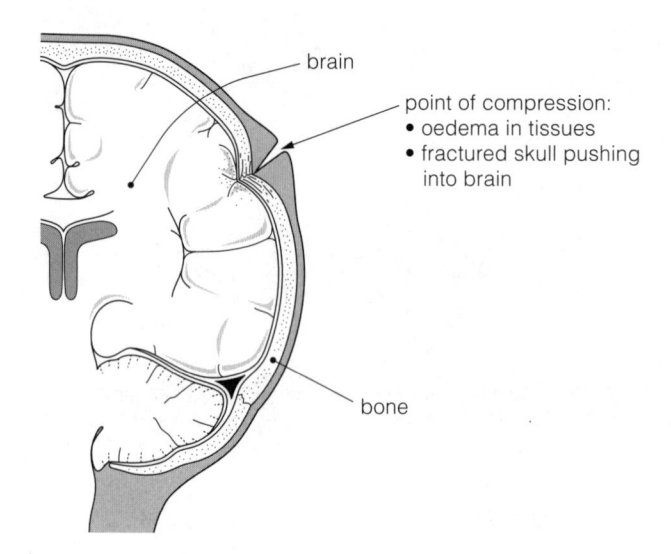

Fig. 1.3 *Skull fracture compressing brain, causing haemorrhage and cerebral damage*

Contre-coup brain injury occurs at the point opposite impact. At the point of impact the brain is compressed and the opposite pole of the brain experiences a negative pressure leading to injury here as well.

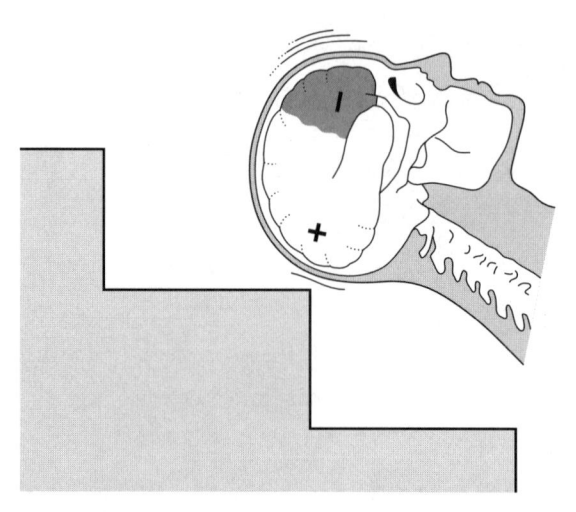

Fig. 1.4 *Contre-coup brain injury*

rest of the body. Internal organs such as the aorta, liver, mesentery and others, which are only partly fixed to the body wall, may continue to move once the body wall has actually stopped. This may result in tearing of structures at points of fixity, such as in the upper descending thoracic aorta, or compression against decelerated tissues, such as the liver against the abdominal wall (Fig. 1.5).

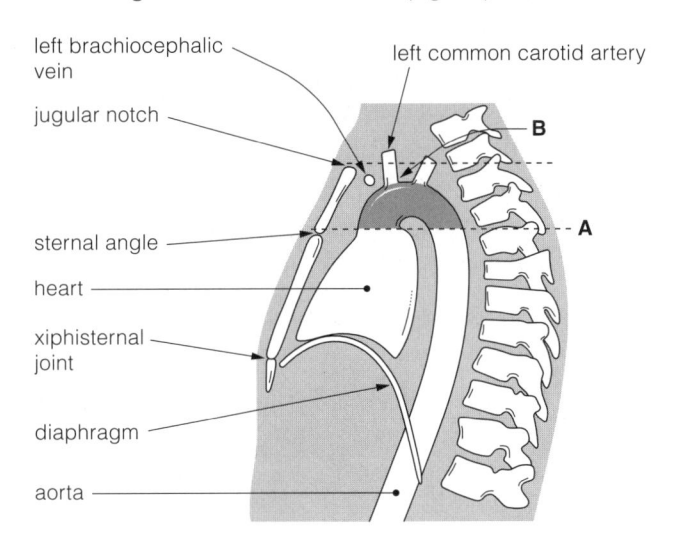

A lateral view of the chest. The aorta below point **A** is *fixed* to the posterior wall of the thorax. It is semi-fixed at the great vessels **B**. When the body decelerates and the free part of the aorta (shaded) continues to move, it may partially or completely tear.

Fig. 1.5 *Thoracic aorta*

Another consequence of body deceleration is the abnormal deformation of bones and joints. For example, the mid-point of the lower leg may be stopped by an object such as the dashboard of a car but the lower portion continues to move, resulting in a fracture to the tibia and fibula (Fig. 1.6). Hyperflexion or hyperextension of the spinal column is also commonly related to deceleration trauma and this can lead to a variety of fractures and spinal cord damage (Fig. 1.7).

In many cases of blunt injury, such as that suffered by the driver of a motor vehicle involved in a head-on collision, there is a combination of the two mechanisms. Direct compression from a steering wheel to the epigastrium may result in rupture of the pancreas, duodenum, stomach or spleen, with possible spinal hyperflexion and fracture leading to spinal cord damage. The rest of the body decelerating may result in thoracic

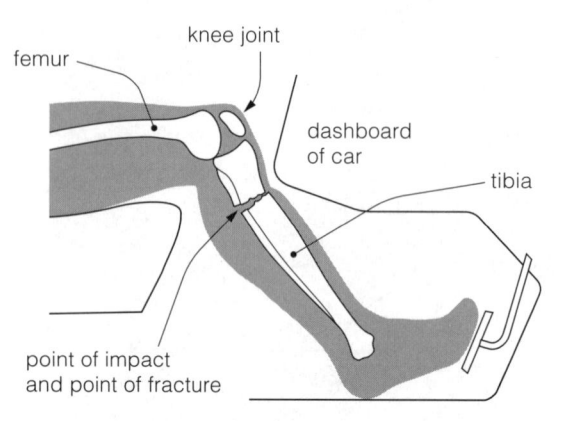

Fig. 1.6 *Fracture occurring at the point of impact where the distal part of the limb continues to move after the proximal part stops*

aortic rupture, cervical spine hyperflexion with further spinal cord trauma and long-bone fractures.

While many of the features described above relate to major trauma, a set of basic principles emerges for this type of injury. Whether major or minor, it can be said that blunt injuries:

- burst tissues raggedly
- contuse tissues and lead to contamination by any substance between the impact and the tissue
- cause compression or deformity to deeper structures
- may be associated with injuries to other body parts

It is these principles, then, that must be borne in mind when assessing injuries of this type.

Kinetic energy injury—open (penetrating)

While less common than blunt trauma there is an increasing incidence of penetrating injuries in Australia. They may be as simple as standing on a nail or as complex as multiple high-velocity bullet wounds. The main differentiating factor is the velocity of the injury. Low-velocity wounds are anything up to the speed of a small-calibre rifle, such as a .22 calibre, and mainly cause damage in the line of the penetration (Fig. 1.8). Higher-velocity projectiles are more dangerous as they cause wide cavitation due to the pressure wave that is created during their passage through tissue (Fig.1.9). Cavitation causes damage to, and devascularisation of, nearby tissues. While somewhat variable the average diameter of the cavitation is about thirty times the diameter of the projectile.

Basic Surgical Skills

(a) The two common modes of cervical spine trauma

hyperextension   hyperflexion

(b)

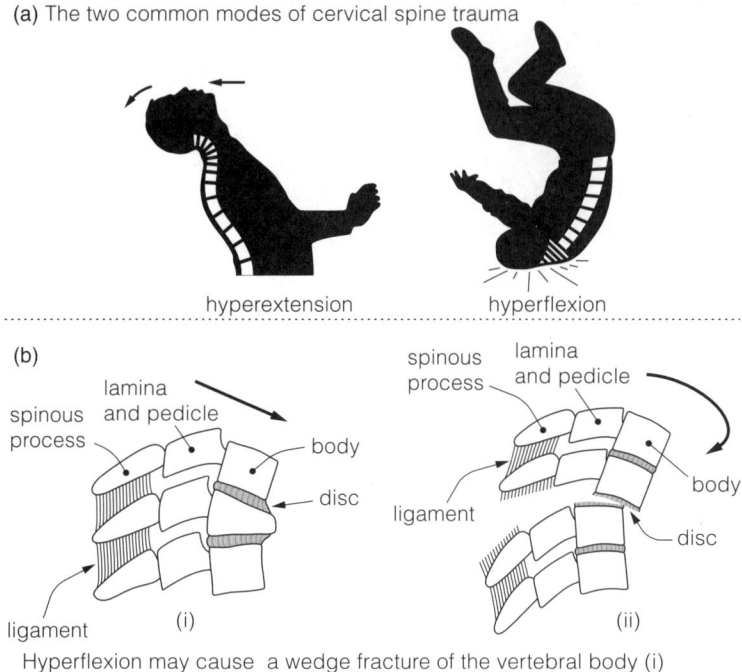

Hyperflexion may cause a wedge fracture of the vertebral body (i) or complete ligamentous and intervertebral joint disruption with partial or complete dislocation (ii). Cord damage is common in both scenarios.

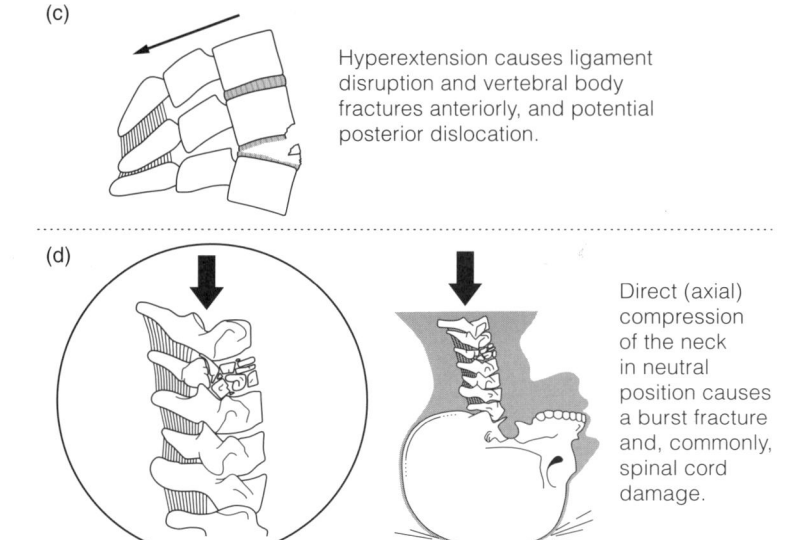

(c) Hyperextension causes ligament disruption and vertebral body fractures anteriorly, and potential posterior dislocation.

(d) Direct (axial) compression of the neck in neutral position causes a burst fracture and, commonly, spinal cord damage.

Fig. 1.7 *Cervical spine hyperflexion and hyperextension leading to spinal cord damage*

The basic principles of wound management

The basic principles of wound management

Table 1.2 Mechanisms of wound causation

Causative factor	Mechanism	Ramifications	Examples
Kinetic energy—closed	• direct crush or compression • shearing force • blast injury	• internal disruption of tissues • haemorrhage • visceral rupture • bony fractures • occult injuries deep or elsewhere	1. A direct steering wheel injury to the epigastrium may result in duodenal, gastric, splenic or hepatic disruption. 2. A limb caught under a vehicle wheel may have skin sheared away from deeper tissues by rotational forces. 3. A cricket ball hit into the close fielder's forehead may lacerate skin, fracture skull and cause contre-coup brain injury.
Kinetic energy—open	• direct penetration of tissues by incision, tear or burst • low versus high velocity	• low velocity penetration causes disruption of all tissues in the line of the wound • high velocity penetration causes wide internal cavitation with little skin damage. This may lead to major tissue disruption, bleeding, visceral rupture and even fractures at some distance from the point of entry	1. Broken beer glass laceration to the hand may damage digital nerves, vessels and tendons deep to the site. 2. Stab wound to right-hand side of chest may penetrate lung, diaphragm and liver. 3. High-velocity bullet wound to the thigh will disrupt muscle widely, fracture the femur and may disrupt nerves and vessels causing distal ischaemia to the limb.
Thermal energy—hot or cold	• direct physical contact • radiant heat	• variable depth of tissue destruction • underlying structure damage	1. Superficial burn causes erythema with blisters and complete healing with little scarring.

The basic principles of wound management

	• superheated substances • heat causes coagulative necrosis • cold causes ischaemia or tissue freezing	• special burns: – respiratory, ocular and genital • other occult injuries related to the thermal source such as blast injuries or fractures from falls	2. Partial thickness burn results in partial dermal destruction with spared islets of skin and healing with variable scarring. Skin grafting may be required. 3. Full thickness burn results in complete skin destruction and may damage deep fascia, muscle, bone and neurovascular structures. Will require grafting and will scar.
Chemical energy—corrosive	• acidic or alkaline • liquid or solid (crystalline)	• coagulates and kills contact tissues with sloughing, the possibility of infection and long-term scarring with wound contracture	1. Acid splash burns to eyes. 2. Caustic soda (alkali) ingestion causes oesophageal mucosal sloughing and long-term stricturing.
Electrical energy	• direct contact with source • point of exit (earth)	• looks small but is extensive and deep entry and exit points with damage between • follows tissue planes or neurovascular bundles	1. Shock to arm, from 240V a.c., can travel along vessels through heart and cause cardiac arrest. 2. A high-voltage shock to the body, earthed through the leg, can cause muscle necrosis, nerve damage, vessel coagulation and subsequent limb infarction.
Ionising radiation	• x-rays • radioactive substances	• burning of skin and deep damage • damage to replicating cells, e.g. haemopoietic, gut • induction of cancers • long-term inflammation and impaired healing	1. Breast x-ray therapy can burn the skin and cause late osteonecrosis of the clavicle and ribs. 2. Prolonged x-ray exposure to the neck increases the risk of thyroid cancers.

Source: Compilation assisted by information from Sabiston's Textbook of Surgery, 15th edn, WB Saunders Co, Philadelphia 1997

Basic Surgical Skills

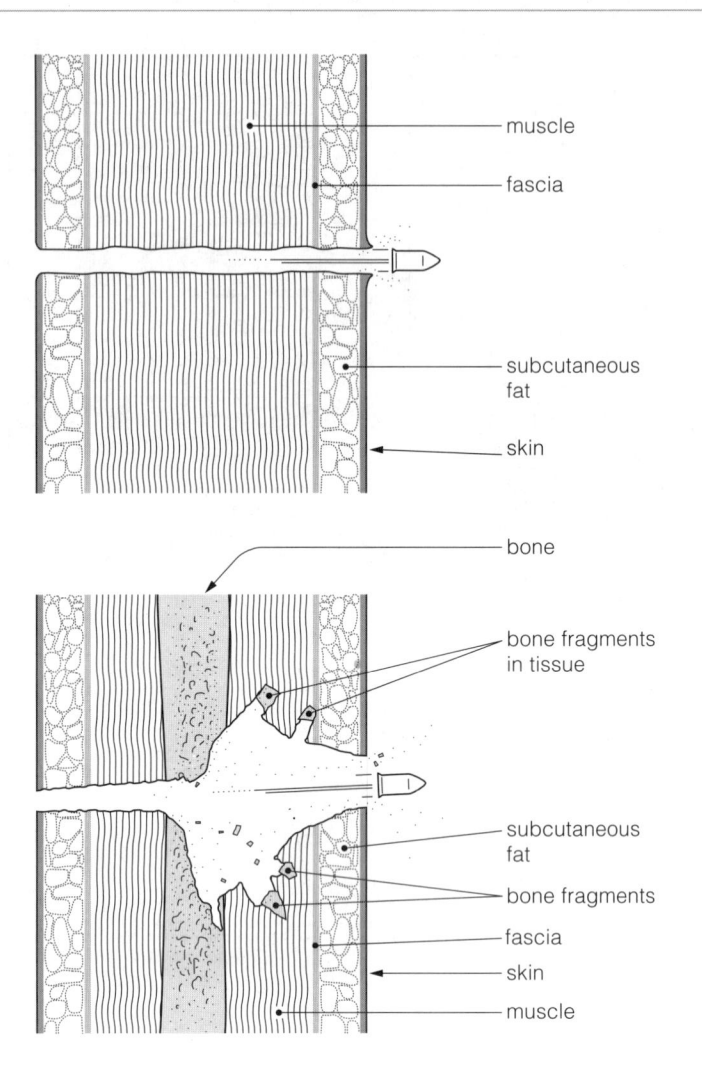

Damage is caused in the line of penetration only. This can be worsened if a bone is fractured and the bone fragments cause damage, or if the bullet itself fragments.

Fig. 1.8 *Tissue injury caused by low-velocity penetrating trauma*

Most penetrating wounds seen in the emergency department will be low-velocity, accidental puncture or incision wounds which are frequently contaminated. *Unless obviously superficial it must be assumed that all deeper structures in the line of the wound are involved.* Examination of distal motor and neurovascular function may suggest which

Basic Surgical Skills

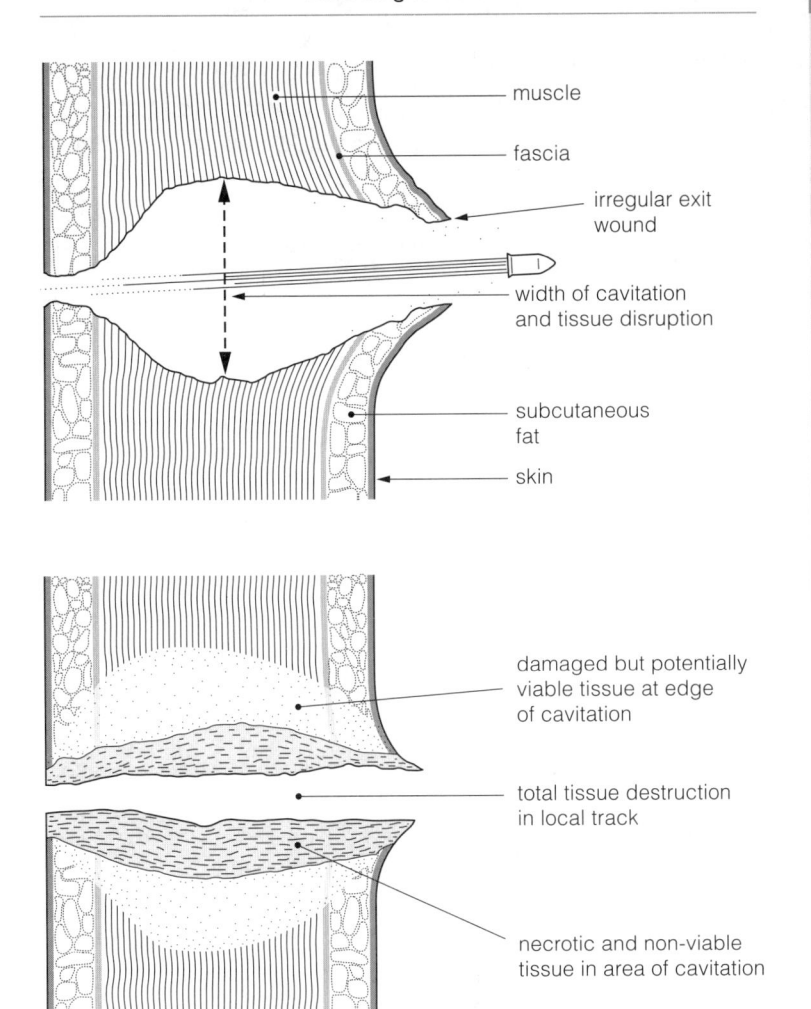

There is widespread damage due to tissue cavitation with high-velocity projectiles.

Fig. 1.9 *Tissue and organ damage caused by high-velocity penetrating trauma*

structures are damaged but partial injury to these may not be detectable. For example, a three-quarters lacerated tendon will function normally with gentle examination but will rupture a week later when stressed. In general, then, exploration to exclude damage to deep structures and to perform wound toilet is almost mandatory in these wounds.

High-velocity projectile wounds are not dealt with in this book.

Thermal energy injury

Thermal injury may be caused by either heat or cold. Dry heat or friction causes a *burn*, moist heat causes a *scald*, prolonged exposure to a cold wet environment causes *chilblains* or *trenchfoot* and actual freezing of tissues by cold causes *frostbite*. While similar in outcome the pathophysiology of heat and cold injuries differs greatly.

Heat injury

The pathology of a heat injury (burn or scald) is a coagulative necrosis of epidermis and dermis to various depths. The depth of this necrosis is the basis for burns classification and the descriptive terms of *first-degree*, *second-degree* and *third-degree* (Fig. 1.10).

A first-degree burn involves part or all of the epidermis. It is caused by a mild heat source such as the sun, or short exposure to a more immediate heat source such as a flame or steam. The injury is always intensely erythematous due to underlying vasodilation and the epidermis either is dry or has small blisters. Involved skin is painful and tender and retains all sensory functions. Infection is rare and healing occurs within a week with no scarring.

A second-degree burn necroses a variable depth of dermis, but not so deeply that it destroys all structures that contain epidermal cells. It is caused by sustained contact with a heat source or chemical. Hair follicles and glandular structures (sebaceous and sweat) are left partially intact and it is the cells lining these, as well as the edges of the burn, that provide the basis for re-epithelialisation. The area appears pink and mottled due to the depth of necrosed tissue overlying the dilated vessels below the burn. Large blisters and copious fluid loss in regions of de-epithelialisation are common. These injuries are intensely painful but, if deep, may lose pinprick sensation. Healing is much slower than in a first-degree burn and there is a moderate risk of infection. Scarring is also common and more severe second-degree burns will require pressure garments or special dressings to reduce this. Occasionally, skin grafting is required but most burns will heal autonomously in two to five weeks. Rehabilitation may be required, as may revisional scar surgery, if contractures prove troublesome.

A third-degree, or full thickness, burn necroses the entire dermis and variable amounts of deeper tissues. Prolonged exposure to the heat source or chemical, extremely high temperatures or high-voltage electrical contact are required to cause this level of destruction.

Basic Surgical Skills

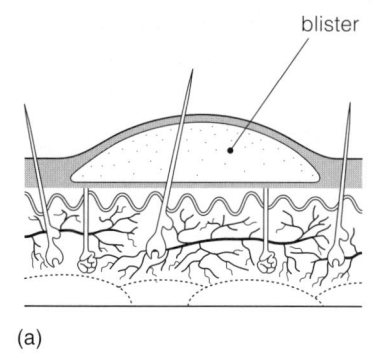

blister

Superficial, or 1st degree, burns affect only the epidermis and result in blistering. These heal themselves in most cases.

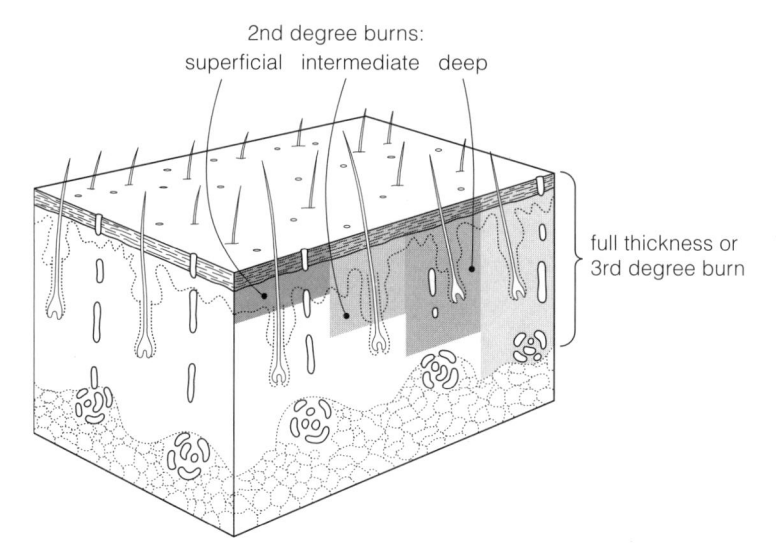

(a)

2nd degree burns: superficial intermediate deep

full thickness or 3rd degree burn

(b) Deeper burns

The deeper the burn the less likely it is to heal. All but the deepest 2nd degree burn will heal. Deep 2nd degree and 3rd degree burns usually require skin grafting.

Fig. 1.10 *Burn thickness/depth*

All epithelium-containing elements are destroyed and therefore spontaneous healing cannot occur. The burn looks pale and marbled due to the depth of injury and vessel thrombosis within it. There is little or no pain (unless there is a zone of lesser-degree burn around it) and all sensory functions of the skin are lost.

Tissue burned this severely is not distensible and, especially if it is a circumferential burn on a limb or torso, underlying tissue pressures may rise due to accumulating inflammatory oedema. If the increase is great enough to prevent blood flow (and hence oxygen delivery) at a microcirculatory level a limb compartment syndrome occurs. In the torso a lack of skin stretch may restrict ventilatory capacity. This situation requires urgent incision of the burned area (escharotomy) and sometimes of the underlying deep fascia (fasciotomy) to relieve or prevent a compartment syndrome and limb ischaemia, or to improve ventilation.

In all third-degree burns the risk of infection is high. Complete excision of the burn followed by skin grafting is routinely used to achieve rapid healing, but scarring is common. The use of pressure garments, revisional scar surgery and rehabilitation is very common.

The patient with cutaneous burns must be examined closely to exclude other injuries. Blunt and penetrating trauma may occur as part of the situation that led to the burn and signs of this must be looked for specifically. There are also special types of burn, such as respiratory burns, ocular burns and genital burns which require the intervention of a specialised practitioner. Assessment of the amount of skin surface area that has been burnt is approximated by the 'rule of nines' (Fig. 1.11).

Table 1.3 outlines the characteristics of burns.

Cold injury

The final effect of cold injury is very similar to that caused by heat—that is, tissue necrosis. Unlike heat, however, it is not a coagulative process from the start. As with heat injury there are levels of severity but they are not classified as strictly as burns.

Mild cold injury is called *pernio* or *chilblains*. These occur on unprotected body parts exposed to a dry source of cold that is above freezing point. Local ulceration, blistering and haemorrhage may occur. The area usually appears cyanosed.

Exposure to a wet cold source that is above freezing point, such as immersion of feet in cold water for one to several days, results in the phenomenon of *trenchfoot*. *Immersion foot* is a similar injury caused by prolonged (days to weeks) exposure to water that is not cold enough to cause trenchfoot. The affected regions appear gangrenous and are usually anaesthetic. The pathology of both is very similar and is due to microvascular endothelial injury, capillary stasis and vascular occlusion. Superficial gangrene may appear impressive but deep tissue loss is usually minimal.

Basic Surgical Skills

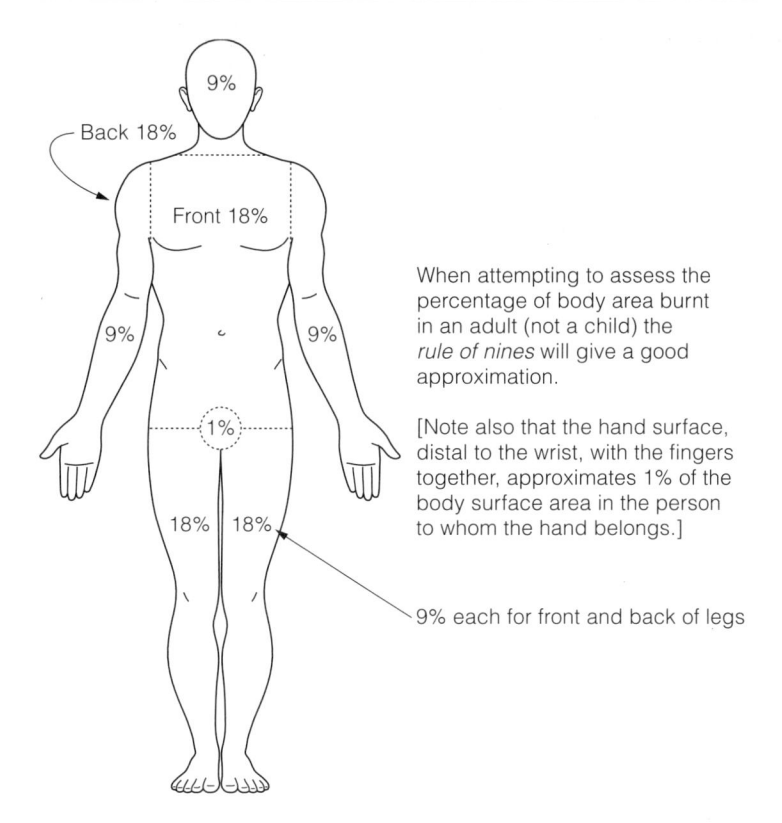

When attempting to assess the percentage of body area burnt in an adult (not a child) the *rule of nines* will give a good approximation.

[Note also that the hand surface, distal to the wrist, with the fingers together, approximates 1% of the body surface area in the person to whom the hand belongs.]

9% each for front and back of legs

Fig. 1.11 *Rule of nines (adult)*

Frostbite is caused by actual freezing of body tissues. The extent of damage is increased by rapidity of freezing and duration of freezing. Pathologically, the injury of frostbite is caused by the combination of freezing and subsequent thawing. Intracellular ice crystallisation, cellular dehydration and microvascular thrombosis begin the process which worsens as the tissue is reheated. There are four levels of frostbite severity (see Table 1.4). Thawing tissue loses protein-rich fluid which increases tissue pressure. Local vasoconstriction also increases (paradoxically) to be at its greatest when tissue temperature reaches 15° Celsius. Both these factors may worsen tissue damage.

Warming is an essential part of treatment although, at least in the short term, it may appear to worsen the injury. Hence, early surgical intervention is not recommended as significant amounts of potentially viable tissue may be removed. Once it is certain that all salvageable tissue has recovered then the smallest possible debridement of tissue

Table 1.3 Characteristics of burns

	First-degree (superficial)	Second-degree (partial thickness)	Third-degree (full thickness)
Cause	• Ultraviolet light (sun) • Short-term exposure to steam, radiant source or hot object	• Longer exposure to steam, hot liquid or object, radiant source or chemical	• Prolonged exposure to hot liquid or object, radiant source or chemical • Contact with high-voltage electricity
Depth	• Epidermal	• Low to mid dermis	• Deep dermis and subcutaneous tissues
Appearance	• Erythematous • Dry or small blisters	• Mottled pink • Large blisters or weeping areas	• Dry and pale with vessel thrombosis (marbled) • May be charred • Deep tissue loss or wet necrosis with chemicals or electricity
Sensation	• Painful with intact pressure and pinprick	• Very painful with intact pressure sensation but potential loss of pinprick if quite deep	• Anaesthetic surface with no intact sensation
Course	• Heals spontaneously • Minimal infection risk • Within 1 week • Minimal scarring	• Most heal spontaneously but occasionally may require grafting • Moderate infection risk • Within 2–5 weeks • Minimal to severe scarring	• May require escharotomy, fasciotomy and surgical management of damaged deeper structures • Always requires skin grafting • High infection risk • Healing time related to severity and scarring • Severe scarring common
Outcome	• Normal tissue	• Occasional contractures and unsightly scars • Scar-reducing pressure garments or dressings sometimes required • Some rehabilitation of limbs and patient may be required	• Flexure and other contractures commonly require surgical treatment • Long-term use of pressure garments • Rehabilitation need based on severity and extent

Source: Compilation assisted by information from *Sabiston's Textbook of Surgery*, 15th edn, WB Saunders Co, Philadelphia 1997

Basic Surgical Skills

Table 1.4 Frostbite severity

Four levels of frostbite severity based on appearance after thawing

- **First-degree**
  Very superficial freezing
  Hyperemia, oedema and minimal necrosis

- **Second-degree**
  Partial thickness injury
  Hyperemia, rapid oedema and large blisters
  Necrosis present
  Sensation intact

- **Third-degree**
  Full thickness skin injury
  Pale with slow-onset oedema
  Eventual necrosis
  Sensation lost

- **Fourth-degree**
  Full skin thickness and deep tissues
  Limb infarction
  Requires amputation

Source: Compilation assisted by information from *Sabiston's Textbook of Surgery*, 15th edn, WB Saunders Co., Philadelphia 1997

---

may be undertaken. In the long term, any of the more severe cold injuries can lead to paraesthesia, cold intolerance, muscle weakness, pain on weight bearing and acrocyanosis. Further discussion regarding the treatment of thermal injury may be found in specialised texts.

Table 1.5 summarises the characteristics of cold injury.

Chemical injury

Many chemical agents cause damage to living tissues and have this effect through a number of mechanisms. These include heat liberation from chemical reactions, liquefaction by strong alkalis, delipidation by petrochemicals and vesicle formation by various gases. The severity of damage is related to such factors as the amount of chemical, its concentration and the duration of contact. Initial treatment is by

The basic principles of wound management

Table 1.5 Characteristics of cold injury

	Chilblains	Trenchfoot	Frostbite
Cause	• Exposure to dry cold above freezing • Vascular cause	• Exposure to cold wet conditions • Vascular cause	• Freezing of tissues • Ice crystals, dehydration and vasospasm
Depth	• Superficial	• Superficial tissues with occasional deep tissue involvement	• Any depth of tissue but is classified according to four levels (see Table 1.4) • Recovery may occur in much of the involved tissue
Appearance	• Small ulcers, blisters and bleeding with local cyanosis	• Macerated and gangrenous tissues widespread on foot and lower leg	• Dry, desquamated, pale, grey and gangrenous appearance
Sensation	• Painful with intact normal sensory function	• Anaesthetic initially • Long-term paraesthesia, cold intolerance and pain with weight bearing may occur	• Anaesthetic initially • Long-term paraesthesia, cold intolerance and pain with weight bearing may occur
Course	• Rapid healing	• Slow healing of most tissue with some superficial (and occasionally deep) tissue loss	• Slow recovery of affected tissue depending on severity • Final demarcation usually much less than initially apparent injury
Outcome	• Normal tissue	• Some tissue loss and scarring	• Variable tissue loss by surgical debridement after final demarcation

Source: Compilation assisted by information from *Sabiston's Textbook of Surgery*, 15th edn, WB Saunders Co. Philadelphia 1997

copious and prolonged irrigation with water. In a very few instances specific solvents or antidotes are required but this decision should be left to specialist treatment facilities. At times early excision is required to minimise local damage.

Certain special cases also occur. In the case of gas exposure respiratory damage may occur and should be suspected. Chemical ocular injuries also need copious irrigation and early consultation with an ophthalmologist.

Electrical injury

Electrical current causes direct tissue injury by conversion to thermal energy at the site of entry and along planes of conduction. This phenomenon is a function of *current density* (i.e. current flow and voltage drop per unit of cross-sectional area). Unlike direct heat injury, however, the deeper tissues cool more slowly than the superficial and are more liable to sustain a greater injury.

The entry wound is usually heavily charred and, at low voltages (less than 1000 V), the increased electrical resistance created by this will prevent further current flow. At high voltages this is not true and the current will continue to flow, causing damage to deeper structures.

The major injuries from high-voltage shocks occur in limbs, with muscle and other deep tissue effectively being 'cooked' by the liberated heat. This leads to myoglobinuria and renal failure which may be further compounded by the failure to appreciate correctly the amount of fluid resuscitation required. Hyperkalaemia may also occur as a consequence of tissue damage and acute renal failure. Increases in tissue pressure will lead to a compartment syndrome and this requires urgent fasciotomy to preserve blood flow to any viable local and distal tissue.

Other consequences of high-voltage shocks include cardiac arrest and rhythm disturbances, central and peripheral neurological injury, visceral injury, spinal compression fractures and late haemorrhage. These should be watched for and patients frequently reassessed during their inpatient stay.

Ionising radiation injury

While radiation is an uncommon source of acute injury an understanding of the biologic basis of radiation damage completes a knowledge of the major mechanisms of tissue injury. In essence, radiation emits energy as it passes through tissue. The amount of energy released varies with the type of radiation source and the tissue being traversed. This energy ionises molecules and starts a chain of biochemical events that leads to the damage of DNA, RNA, cellular fibres and membranes. The effects of this include cell death, chromosomal rearrangements and point mutations. These changes are variably reversible. Individual cells appear to be more sensitive if they divide frequently (e.g. haemopoietic stem cells) and less sensitive if they don't (e.g. nerve cells).

Local tissue effects of radiation endarteritis, with progressive devascularisation and fibrosis, worsen the transfer of nutrients to irradiated regions. This impairs wound healing and increases the rate of wound breakdown in these areas. Late manifestations of radiation injury may include radiation-induced malignancies, radiation osteonecrosis and underlying organ damage (e.g. heart, lungs and gut). Very high doses of radiation, such as those received in nuclear explosions or accidents, cause widespread proliferative cell death. This in turn breaks down host barriers, such as the gut, and defences, such as the immune cell system, and leads to eventual demise of the organism.

The pathology of wound healing

Understanding the type, mechanism and ramifications of a wound comprises the first step in the ability to manage it effectively. A sound knowledge of wound healing and factors that affect this, in the individual patient, is equally important for the adequate assessment of a traumatic wound.

Wound healing

The repair of any soft tissue relies on:
- the body generating capillaries and collagen on both sides of the wound
- this collagen cross-linking with wound-edge collagen and new collagen
- the wound contracting in size
- the unaligned, cross-linked collagen maturing into regularly arranged bundles (a scar) to provide the healed wound with strength
- epithelial regrowth across the defect

While the actual process is identical, no matter how the wound is managed, three modes of wound healing are described. *First intention healing*, or primary closure, describes the reparative process with the wound closed and the edges brought together (Fig. 1.12). *Second intention healing* describes repair when the wound is left open and it slowly heals from the base up (Fig. 1.13). A combination of these two methods, *delayed primary closure*, relies on the wound initially remaining open, beginning granulation, and the edges subsequently being closed together to speed the healing process.

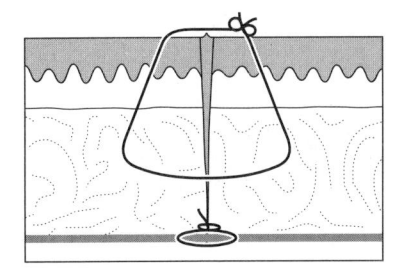

(a) All layers approximated with sutures and narrow gap filled with fibrin.

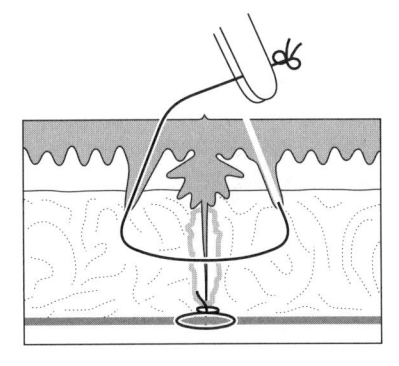

(b) Removal of skin sutures several days later. Epithelial growth into dermis at suture tracks and wound.

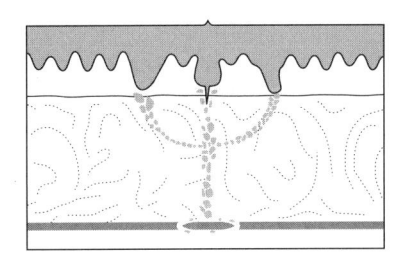

(c) Weeks later the epithelial plugs are disintegrating and fine scars develop in the wound and suture tracks. Absorbable sutures disintegrate.

Fig. 1.12 *First intention healing, or primary closure*

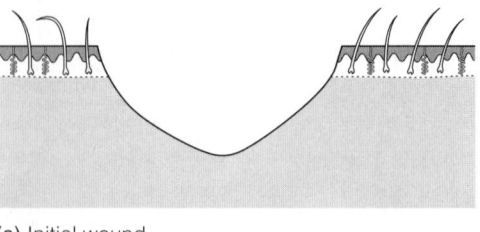

(a) Initial wound

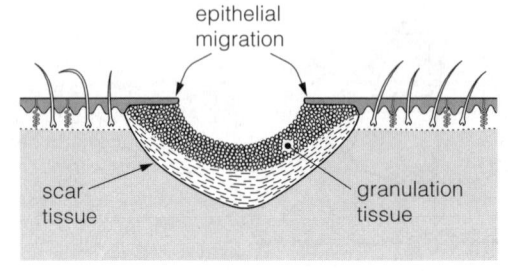

(b) Simultaneous development of granulation tissue and epithelial migration. Wound contraction causes the gap to reduce.

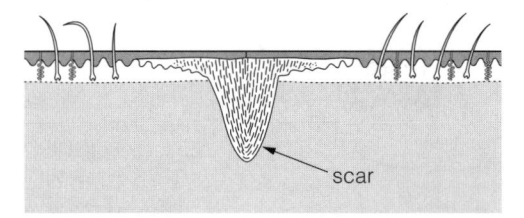

(c) Final result is scar contracture and epithelial cover devoid of skin appendages or rete ridges.

Fig. 1.13 *Second intention healing*

Second intention healing

A description of the healing process of an open wound supplies the basic description of the healing for all wounds. The beginning of this process is filling of the open defect with clot and exudate. Drying of the surface provides a crust to cover the moist depths of the wound. In the moist region, collagenolysis and digestion of tissue by phagocytic white blood cells is the body's own form of wound debridement. Subsequently, capillary loops grow, from the edges of the wound, into a matrix of white blood cells, mucopolysaccharides and fibroblast which produces collagen. This is called granulation tissue. Specially differentiated actin and myosin containing fibroblasts (myofibroblasts) aid the healing process by causing wound contraction. Gradually the collagen, which is both types 1 and 3, cross-links and forms the basis of the scar. Epithelium migrates from the edges of the wound to cover this tissue. Over a period of six to twelve months the collagen in the scar realigns (matures), type 3 collagen is lost and more type 1 is laid down, the scar thins and the hyperaemic, capillary-rich scar tissue pales as vessels diminish in size and number.

First intention healing

First intention healing occurs by virtually the same processes, but only in that minute gap between accurately opposed wound edges. Fibrinous adhesion between the surfaces occurs by about 24 hours but there is little strength until true healing begins. As in other wounds, granulation tissue grows in and collagen is laid down. Contraction, scar formation, re-epithelialisation and scar maturation also occur. The difference between first and second intention healing is, therefore, quantitative rather than qualitative.

In Figure 1.14 the graph illustrates the increase in wound strength over time.

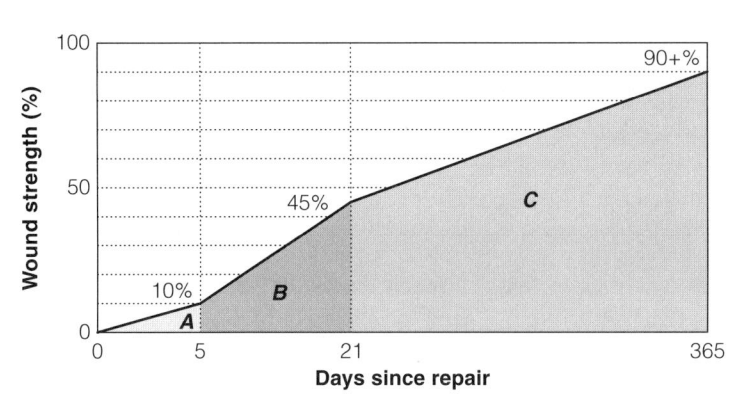

A *Lag phase* **Days 1–4**. Inflammation and phagocyte debridement. Initial collagenolysis (may be marked in bowel) and assembly of components for collagen synthesis. Strength mainly dependent on sutures.

B *Proliferative phase* **Days 5–21**. Fibroblasts lay down a collagen lattice in a ground substance.
Rapid increase of wound strength to about 30–50%.
Period during which sutures are usually removed.

C *Remodelling phase* **Days 22–1 year**. Process of constant absorption and replacement of collagen in the wound along lines of stress. Strength increases to virtually 100% over this period.

Fig. 1.14 *Healing processes and wound strength*

Factors influencing wound healing

The factors that affect the healing of wounds can be divided into three categories—local, general and technical. If we look at each of these categories in relation to the healing process the effect of each factor must be to cause mechanical disruption, necrosis, reduction in local collagen, an inhibition of new collagen formation or a combination of these. The outcome may range from a minor wound infection through to non-healing and major dehiscence of the wound.

Local factors

Ischaemia

Ischaemia is the lack of blood (and hence nutrient and oxygen) supply to living tissue. In a healing wound this may be due to:

- inadequate vascular inflow to the repaired tissue because of vessel ligation, peripheral vascular disease or generalised hypotension
- the presence of already dead tissue at the wound edge
- overly tight or closely spaced sutures preventing flow through capillaries at the wound's edge
- tension on the wound edges leading to high tissue pressures and increased tension on sutures, thereby preventing flow

Individually, or in combination, these factors reduce blood flow at the healing edges of the wound. This reduces white blood cell and fibroblast inflow, oxygen and nutrient supply and capillary ingrowth. Failure to heal with subsequent wound disruption, wound infection or frank necrosis of wound edges are the final outcomes of this problem.

Ischaemia is prevented by ensuring tissue is loosely apposed and sutures are not tied tightly. The need for excessive tension in closure should prompt consideration of grafting or healing by secondary intention.

Tension

If a tissue defect requires excessive amounts of force to draw the edges together, and retain that position, there is significant risk of wound tension. Wounds in areas of skin mobility or with large amounts of skin loss are particularly prone to this. The resultant mechanical distraction forces lead to ischaemia due to tightening of sutures, the tearing out of sutures and increased deep dead space. Elimination of tension by the use of grafts and flaps, postoperative splinting to prevent wound movement or allowing healing by secondary intention will lessen or prevent these problems.

Dead space
The presence of a cavity deep in the wound allows for collection of blood and serous fluid. This provides an ideal culture medium for bacteria and predisposes to infection. Attention to accurate wound closure will reduce wound dead space.

Foreign bodies and contamination
The presence of extraneous foreign material, dead tissue and a large amount (inoculum) of bacteria all increase the risk of infection and wound disruption. Wounds in 'dirty regions' (e.g. groin and natal cleft), long duration of contamination, bacterial virulence and antibiotic resistance compound this problem. Prevention is by adequate debridement, wound lavage and the use of antibiotics in certain circumstances.

Wound infection
Wound infection is a problem in contaminated wounds, ischaemic wounds and those in which haematoma or fluid collections have occurred. With the accompanying local inflammatory response, collagenolysis increases and tissue pressure elevates. These can combine to cause further ischaemia and retard the healing process. Prevention or early treatment of wound infection by a combination of antibiotics and drainage can save major wound and patient complications.

Haematoma
The presence of a wound haematoma predisposes to infection and subsequent wound complications. Inadequate haemostasis, bleeding due to the relaxation of vessel spasm, late bleeding in wound infection or patient anticoagulation by drugs or disseminated intravascular coagulopathy are the major reasons for haemorrhage. Close attention to haemostasis and relevant patient factors will minimise the risk of this.

Local trauma
Damage to tissues may contuse and render them partially or totally ischaemic. This may provide a nidus for infection. Local trauma also increases the inflammatory response in a way similar to sepsis, thereby promoting collagenolysis (especially related to gastrointestinal anastomosis). It may also increase the rate of sepsis. Care in operative management and wide debridement will minimise this.

Chronic tissue factors
Local tissue problems such as chronic lymphoedema, chronic ischaemia, venous hypertension and past scarring can all contribute to poor

wound healing. Little can be done for these conditions other than the use of assiduous techniques and optimisation of other factors.

Sutures
Tightly tied sutures can cause ischaemia and wound-edge necrosis. Certain suture materials, such as silk, cause an increased inflammatory response and may increase wound infection rates and collagenolysis. Sutures may also 'cut out'. Gentle but firm knots and minimal wound tension will minimise this factor.

Irradiation
With the modern trend of preoperative irradiation in certain disorders (e.g. rectal cancer) tissue healing may be impaired due to the fibrosis and microangiopathy associated with this treatment. Postoperative radiotherapy may also increase the incidence of wound complications.

Conclusion
As can be seen from the descriptions above, all local factors can contribute directly to poor healing. Interestingly, each may also contribute to creating or worsening other factors. Resolution of only one of these problems, then, may have far-reaching implications in reducing or preventing a wide range of other adverse factors, thereby avoiding an adverse wound outcome.

General factors
The following general factors may all play a part in retarding the healing of any wound because of their effect on local factors as well as their endogenous effects on collagen synthesis and immune function. Individually, they may cause only minor problems but many patients present with a number of these factors and do, predictably, quite poorly. The factors include:

- age/medical conditions—e.g. diabetes, renal failure, hepatic failure, respiratory failure, immunodeficiencies, obesity
- anaemia/blood loss
- shock/hypovolaemia/hypoxia
- weight loss/malnutrition (inc. Vit C, Zn, Vit A, proteins etc.)
- major infections/septicaemia
- advanced malignancy
- steroid use

Many of these factors are partially remediable in the perioperative period and particular attention should be paid to identifying and reversing as many of them as possible. In the more severely unwell individual this may entail the use of medical, anaesthetic and intensive care consultation.

Technical factors

These two poorly quantifiable factors—wound evaluation skills and surgical techniques—depend very much on the individual practitioner. Adequacy of initial instruction and appropriate amounts of supervised experience are the only ways to develop the skills to deal appropriately with wounds. Wound evaluation, reflecting the available skills and experience to make decisions for each individual wound, and the technical abilities to deal with the wound surgically are an inseparable combination. In general, they reflect the clinical ability and judgment of an individual at a given time and therefore may differ for the same person over time. It is doubtful, however, that increasing experience equates to better skills and practice, and it is likely that appropriate ability is really a threshold phenomenon.

Table 1.6 lists the factors affecting wound healing.

Table 1.6 Factors affecting wound healing

Class	Factors
Local factors	• Ischaemia • Tension • Dead space • Foreign bodies/contamination • Wound infection • Haematoma • Chronic tissue factors • Local trauma • Sutures • Irradiation
General factors	• Age/comorbidity, e.g. diabetes, renal failure • Anaemia/blood loss • Shock hypovolaemia/hypoxia • Malnutrition—protein and micronutrient • Major infections/septicaemia • Advanced malignancy • Steroid use
Technical factors	• Wound evaluation skills • Surgical techniques

Conclusions

As many of these factors as possible should be identified and reversed, or at least addressed, in order to maximise the rate of healing achieved in adverse conditions. This will usually, but not always, lead to a successful patient outcome. Failure to identify reversible factors by inadequate assessment and understanding is at best inexcusable and will often result in adverse outcomes.

The surgical management of wounds

Before undertaking the responsibility of wound assessment and management, an understanding of wounds, wound healing and factors affecting wound healing is mandatory. Assuming this knowledge, this section aims to provide a basic format for the evaluation of a small, peripheral, traumatic wound and the principles involved in this wound's management. With experience, readers will be able to modify these to suit their own practice and individual situations as required.

The evaluation of more severe wounds, burns of any type and critically injured patients is not dealt with here. This type of global assessment is the province of formal trauma education systems such as the Royal Australasian College of Surgeons Early Management of Severe Trauma (EMST) course and the Advanced Trauma Life Support (ATLS) course of the American College of Surgeons.

Wound evaluation

The evaluation of minor traumatic wounds is based on three main tasks:

1. ascertain the mechanism of injury
2. examine the wound site
3. decide on the method of repair

The first task is to *ascertain the mechanism of injury by taking an accurate history.* In knowing this mechanism, especially the causative implement and angle and depth of penetration, potential sites of concomitant or occult injury can be predicted. Symptoms of deep structure damage such as anaesthesia with nerve damage, inability to move digits with tendon damage, and pain on movement symptomatic of deep compartment penetration must be specifically enquired after. At the same time, factors that may affect the choice of repair or the healing process should be sought.

Secondly, an *assiduous examination of the wound site and deep tissues*, if possible, will allow classification of the wound type and give further clues to the amount of damage suffered by underlying structures. This process must include testing for distal motor and neurovascular competence prior to anaesthetic administration. Examination of involved or adjacent bones and joints, seeking restrictions or excesses of movement in both passive and active ranges, may suggest joint, bone, ligament or tendon damage. Obvious deformity will suggest fracture. If bony damage or foreign body are suspected an x-ray is a useful and justifiable examination.

Thirdly, *a decision regarding the method of repair* must be made. This must take into account wound severity and structures involved, wound size and skin loss and factors that may affect healing. If the wound is a minor, type 1 to 3 injury with no deep involvement and minimal adverse factors, repair should be undertaken in the Emergency Department by an appropriately experienced practitioner.

Large amounts of skin loss, actual or potential involvement of any major structures, uncertainty regarding depth or extent of damage, type 3 or 4 wounds, inexperience, inadequate facilities, the presence of any adverse factors (see section on factors above) or the potential need for complicated rehabilitation all mandate further assessment by an experienced practitioner or inpatient surgical team (see Table 1.7). Acceptable conditions for formal exploration and repair are usually found only in the operating theatre. Optimum lighting, good equipment, experienced assistance and absolute anaesthesia (whether regional or general) provide the surgeon with an environment where all injuries can be dealt with appropriately, thus contributing to a potentially improved outcome for the patient.

Figure 1.15 presents a schema for the management of a minor wound.

Principles of treatment and repair

In repairing an acute traumatic wound there are many basic principles that should be considered. These begin in the decision-making phase and may continue until complete healing of the wound.

Before repair

Closure

Confirm that the decision to close the wound is the correct one. If there is any doubt about skin loss, injuries to other structures,

Basic Surgical Skills

The basic principles of wound management

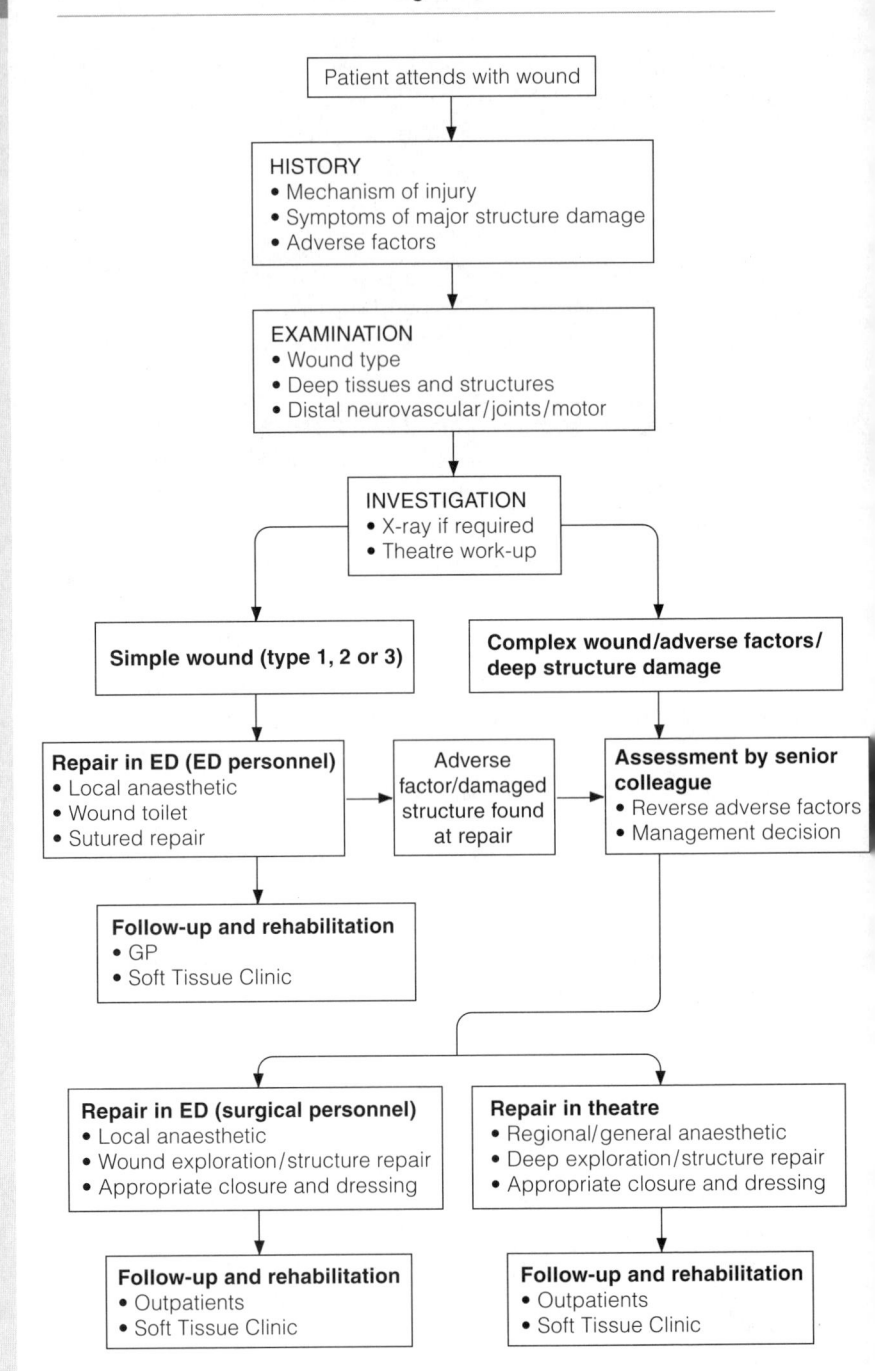

```
Patient attends with wound
          │
          ▼
┌─────────────────────────────────────┐
│ HISTORY                             │
│ • Mechanism of injury               │
│ • Symptoms of major structure damage│
│ • Adverse factors                   │
└─────────────────────────────────────┘
          │
          ▼
┌─────────────────────────────────────┐
│ EXAMINATION                         │
│ • Wound type                        │
│ • Deep tissues and structures       │
│ • Distal neurovascular/joints/motor │
└─────────────────────────────────────┘
          │
          ▼
┌─────────────────────────────────────┐
│ INVESTIGATION                       │
│ • X-ray if required                 │
│ • Theatre work-up                   │
└─────────────────────────────────────┘
       ↙             ↘
┌──────────────────┐   ┌──────────────────────────────┐
│ Simple wound     │   │ Complex wound/adverse factors│
│ (type 1, 2 or 3) │   │ /deep structure damage       │
└──────────────────┘   └──────────────────────────────┘
         │                            │
         ▼                            │
┌──────────────────┐  ┌──────────────┐ ┌──────────────────────┐
│ Repair in ED     │  │ Adverse      │ │ Assessment by senior │
│ (ED personnel)   │─▶│ factor/      │▶│ colleague            │
│ • Local          │  │ damaged      │ │ • Reverse adverse    │
│   anaesthetic    │  │ structure    │ │   factors            │
│ • Wound toilet   │  │ found        │ │ • Management decision│
│ • Sutured repair │  │ at repair    │ └──────────────────────┘
└──────────────────┘  └──────────────┘
         │
         ▼
┌──────────────────────────┐
│ Follow-up and rehabilitation │
│ • GP                     │
│ • Soft Tissue Clinic     │
└──────────────────────────┘
              ↙                    ↘
┌──────────────────────────────┐  ┌──────────────────────────────┐
│ Repair in ED                 │  │ Repair in theatre            │
│ (surgical personnel)         │  │ • Regional/general anaesthetic│
│ • Local anaesthetic          │  │ • Deep exploration/structure │
│ • Wound exploration/         │  │   repair                     │
│   structure repair           │  │ • Appropriate closure and    │
│ • Appropriate closure and    │  │   dressing                   │
│   dressing                   │  │                              │
└──────────────────────────────┘  └──────────────────────────────┘
           │                                  │
           ▼                                  ▼
┌──────────────────────────┐    ┌──────────────────────────┐
│ Follow-up and rehabilitation │ │ Follow-up and rehabilitation │
│ • Outpatients            │    │ • Outpatients            │
│ • Soft Tissue Clinic     │    │ • Soft Tissue Clinic     │
└──────────────────────────┘    └──────────────────────────┘
```

Fig. 1.15 *Management of a minor wound*

Table 1.7 Criteria for seeking expert assessment of wounds

1. Inexperience
2. Large skin loss
3. Demonstrated deep structure injury
4. Suspected or potential deep structure injury
5. Large or complicated wound
6. Type 3 or 4 wound
7. Inadequate facilities for repair
8. Adverse factors—local
    —general
    —technical
9. Rehabilitation required

contamination or any other adverse factors seek the advice of a senior colleague before proceeding.

Explanation and consent

Without doubt one of the most effective methods of medicolegal protection is good communication. In obtaining consent for the repair (or any procedure) four main areas should be discussed:

1. the procedure to be carried out and any other treatment required
2. the alternatives to your treatment plan
3. the benefits of your treatment plan
4. the risks of both your treatment plan and the alternative plans

Further discussion should also describe the planned outcome, ongoing treatment needs, follow-up and plans for rehabilitation. Explanation of potential problems in the postoperative period, how to recognise them and when to present for reassessment are also important for each patient.

Antimicrobials

Antibiotics are thought to make a difference in visibly contaminated and infected wounds and must be given as soon as possible after injury. Penicillin derivatives such as flucloxacillin or dicloxacillin provide staphylococcus cover and penicillin V provides cover for streptococcus and some clostridial species. Erythromycin and cephalexin are oral alternatives for staphylococcus and streptococcus. Enteric flora require a second or third generation cephalosporin, or gentamicin, and metronidazole to cover anaerobes.

Tetanus is an infection by the anaerobic, spore-forming, gram positive bacillus *Clostridium tetani*. It enters the wound as spores and incubates in the warm anaerobic environment of devitalised wound tissue. Tetanus-prone wounds are those that have deep contamination from any external source. Inevitably, the greater the contamination, and the more devitalised the tissues, the greater the risk.

Immunisation against tetanus is now widespread and it is rarely a problem. Those people who have not had a booster in more than five years should be given one. If not immunised for more than ten years a full reimmunisation should be undertaken. In these patients, or patients with an uncertain status, passive immunisation with anti-tetanus immunoglobulin may be required until active immunity is reacquired.

Tetanus, and other clostridial or synergistic infections, such as gas gangrene and necrotising fasciitis, are life-threatening. Diabetes, immunosuppression, peripheral vascular disease and carcinoma may all predispose to these. Adequate debridement, provision of immune prophylaxis, antibiotics and treatment of wounds openly by dressing and redebridement are some of the measures required to prevent necrotising infections.

The repair

There is a set of minimum requirements for safe repair of soft tissue wounds in the emergency department. Adequate light, instruments, anaesthesia, resuscitation facilities and a sterile field are all required. The following considerations bear special mention now but are also dealt with more fully in Chapters 4, 5 and 6. A summary of factors required for good management is found in Table 1.8.

Anaesthesia

If a wound is small or superficial adjacent infiltration of local anaesthesia or a peripheral nerve block is usually adequate. Xylocaine is a rapid-acting anaesthetic for short-term local anaesthesia. The addition of adrenaline prolongs the action slightly and increases the amount able to be used safely. Further information on local anaesthesia is found in Chapter 5 and in the Further Reading section of this chapter.

Wound preparation and the sterile field

Local anaesthesia is best administered early so that gross decontamination with soap and water, antiseptics and a scrubbing brush can be performed before prepping. Skin around the wound site should be

Table 1.8 Factors in wound management

- Antimicrobials
  - —antibiotics
  - —tetanus prophylaxis
- Anaesthesia
- Haemostasis
- Debridement and irrigation
- Wound closure
  - —method
  - —materials
- Immobilisation

widely shaved and prepared to allow wound extension and skin graft harvest if required. As with any surgical procedure a sterile field is mandatory. This is achieved by preparing the wound with antiseptic solutions of povidone iodine or chlorhexidine. Alcohol-based prep solutions are better avoided due to their irritant potential and fire risk. Sterile towels are draped over the unprepared regions and operating table to prevent contamination.

Debridement

Any contaminated wound requires the debridement of dead and devitalised tissues, foreign bodies and contaminating bacteria to prevent infection and necrosis. Excision of the wound margins to various levels will reclassify the wound and must include bone, fascia, muscle, fat, foreign material and skin. Copious irrigation will also help to reduce the volume of bacterial innoculum and prevent further infective complications. Remove as much skin and tissue as necessary to create a 'clean' wound (debridement of 1–2 mm is usually adequate for skin edges) and enough 'dirty' wound tissue to create freely bleeding surfaces. Skin edges should be incised perpendicular to the skin surface to ensure the greatest likelihood of a fine linear scar.

Haemostasis

Tissue that bleeds will generally heal, whereas ischaemic tissue may provide a seat for infection and prevent healing. Uncontrolled wound bleeding, however, may cause a wound haematoma and also predispose to infection or non-healing. All major vessels in the wound should be ligated or electrocauterised. After debridement back to bleeding tissue, the minimal use of diathermy and ligatures may be necessary to restore haemostasis again.

Closure

A decision must be made as to the best method of closure for a wound. In clean wounds, or contaminated wounds that have been surgically converted to clean, direct suture in layers allows first intention healing. If there is any doubt about the viability of tissue, or the risk of infection, closure should not be performed. In this scenario the wound may either be left open and allowed to granulate, healing by second intention, or an ongoing course of wound debridement and later closure may be used. This final method is called *delayed primary closure*. Deep structures such as bone, vessels, nerves or tendons may also require specialised repair or fixation prior to soft tissue or skin closure. Skin grafts and flaps are not considered here.

Choice of suture material

In the modern era we can classify suture material in three ways:

- natural vs synthetic
- absorbable vs non-absorbable
- monofilament vs braided/twisted

Non-absorbable sutures are used for skin (and removed) and for some deep structures such as tendons, vessels and nerve repairs (but not removed). Absorbable sutures are used for deep tissues, membranes and subcuticular skin closure. These are discussed further in Chapter 3.

Dressings and splints

After suturing, tincture of benzoin may be applied to the wound edges and adhesive strips used to take tension off the skin and aid in apposition. Dressing should be non-adherent (e.g. tulle gras or telfa) with gauze over it and a bandage or plastic adhesive dressing. If there has been repair of a deep structure such as a tendon, nerve, vessel or bone, or if the wound is in a mobile region, the wound site should be splinted with a plaster slab or cast. Padded aluminium splints are also available for finger and hand work but are probably less effective.

Table 1.9 gives bandage sizes for various body parts.

After repair

The discharge routine from the emergency department should include the provision of slings or crutches where appropriate, the prescription of antibiotics and analgesics, arrangements for follow-up and rehabilitation. Best posturing and allowed movements, normal course of

Table 1.9 Bandage sizes for body parts

Finger/Hand	2.5 cm
Wrist/Forearm	5.0 cm
Upper arm/Calf	7.5 cm
Thigh	10–15 cm
Head	10–15 cm

healing, variants to be expected during this time, problems to return for and who to consult also need to be discussed. Appropriate work certificates should be provided at this time.

Conclusions

For any practitioner who plans to manage traumatic wounds an understanding of wound type, mechanism and healing are vital. Strict adherence to the basic principles of wound evaluation and repair will inevitably lead to a high rate of both cosmetic and functional wound healing. Unfortunately, failure to perform an adequate assessment of both the patient and the wound, or neglect of the principles of repair, may condemn the patient to a protracted and unsatisfactory course of management.

Further reading

Friedin J & Marshall V. *Illustrated Guide to Surgical Practice*, Churchill Livingstone, Melbourne, 1984. Chap. 1, Wounds—Healing and Management.

McGregor IA. *Fundamental Techniques of Plastic Surgery*, 8th edn, Churchill Livingstone, Edinburgh, 1989. Chap. 1, Wound Care.

Sabiston Jr DC ed. *Sabiston's Textbook of Surgery*, 15th edn, WB Saunders Co., Philadelphia, 1997. Chap. 13, Burns.

Thompson RVS. *Primary Repair of Soft Tissue Injuries*, Melbourne University Press, Melbourne, 1969. Chaps 1–10.

CHAPTER TWO

Surgical instruments and their uses

The ability to undertake increasingly more complex surgical procedures has been mirrored by the development and use of more sophisticated and functional surgical tools. Most new instruments, however, are merely refinements on long-established patterns, with the notable exception of some laparoscopic styles. Suture manufacturers, on the other hand, are constantly involved in the design and testing of newer and better materials. Likewise, new needle materials and shapes (particularly blunt needles for fascia) have changed both practices and patterns of use.

The basic aim of this section of the manual is to provide an easily understood classification of surgical instrumentation, a visual guide to some basic instruments and a description of their common uses. In each subsection representative examples are illustrated. Some eponyms have been used, as they can be useful in differentiating a specific instrument. Unfortunately, the use of eponyms can also cause confusion and difficulty if the specific instrument is not available or the wrong name is used. This may lead to a long and fruitless search of theatre for the item when an acceptable 'generic' alternative is already present on the instrument setup.

In deciding which instruments to present a great number of specialised tools have been overlooked. You will note that there is no coverage of orthopaedic drills or many of the instruments from other surgical specialties. Some exceptions have been made, however, for specialty instruments that are used frequently by general surgeons.

Cutting instruments

The instruments used for cutting tissues have been divided into three groups:

1. Scalpels
2. Scissors
3. Other cutting instruments

Scalpels

Scalpels have been regarded as the traditional tool of the surgeon for centuries. In recent years a two-piece version (permanent handle and disposable blade) has been the standard instrument. The scalpel is used for the deliberate and precise division of structures with the minimum trauma to surrounding tissue. The blade is always sharp (as it can be replaced whenever it seems blunt) and there is a variety of blades and handles available for use. Scalpels can be used to divide skin, connective tissues, muscle, cartilage and viscera. They should not be used on metal or bone.

The scalpel is also traditionally used for incising the peritoneum during a laparotomy as it is tented between two artery forceps. The rationale is that a light touch with the scalpel will make a tiny hole, allow air into the peritoneal cavity and so allow viscera to drop away from the parietal peritoneum. A scissor, on the other hand, could cut structures lying against the peritoneum internally.

The whole length of the blade, not just the tip, should be employed in cutting and it should always be held at $90°$ to the skin surface. For long skin incision, such as in a laparotomy, a large handle and blade (e.g. size 4 handle and 22 blade) are employed. The scalpel should be held like a dinner knife. The handle is placed horizontally 'underhand' between the thumb and middle finger with the ring and little fingers wrapped around its back end. The index finger is placed on the back of the actual blade, towards its base. Incised depth is controlled by a combination of drawing the blade smoothly over the tissues and a constant, firm, downward pressure being exerted on the blade by the forearm (Fig. 4.13a).

For smaller incisions or fine dissection work, such as excising small lesions or dirty wound edges, a small handle and blade (e.g. size 3 handle and 15 blade) should be used. In these instances the scalpel is held more like a pen and most of the movement comes from the hand and fingers. With this grip the surgeon's wrist can be placed against the patient, an instrument or another hand to steady the blade while cutting (Fig. 4.13b).

The ease of cutting with a scalpel is one of its great problems. Inappropriate assessment of a situation may lead to the incision or division of a vital structure (e.g. peripheral nerve). Some simple rules will minimise this risk.

1. Do not cut anything that cannot actually be seen.
2. If the tissue to be divided is superficial to a vital structure, insert an instrument or cutting guide between them.
3. If dissecting near a known structure (e.g. nerve or vessel) cut in the line of the structure to prevent dividing it accidentally.
4. Plan (and mark) your incisions and practise the cut in the air first.
5. If cutting in a deep cavity, time spent improving the access and exposure equates to time saved repairing a potential error.

Scalpel handles

The two most common handles are the Bard Parker style, in sizes 3 and 4. The numbers refer to the size of the attachment point for the blade as well as handle dimensions. Standard handles are straight and flat (Fig. 2.1) but long, curved and octagonal profile handles are all available for special situations.

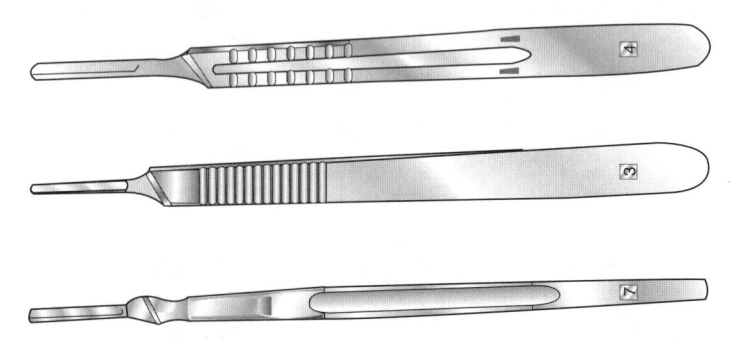

Note the different size heads for attaching the blades to.

Fig. 2.1 *Scalpel handles, sizes 3, 4 and 7*

Scalpel blades

Blades come in various sizes and shapes. The larger ones are used for long incisions in thick skin (e.g. on the trunk) while the smaller and finer blades are used for small, thin skin incisions, dissecting viscera or incising vessels (Figs. 2.2 and 2.3). Special blades are also available for specific areas such as ophthalmology.

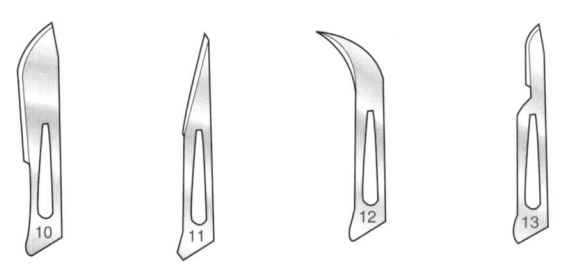

Small scapel blades for fine work are used on a size 3 or 7 handle. Note the hooked 12 blade which can also be used by hand and is designed as a stitch cutter.

Fig. 2.2 *Small scalpel blades*

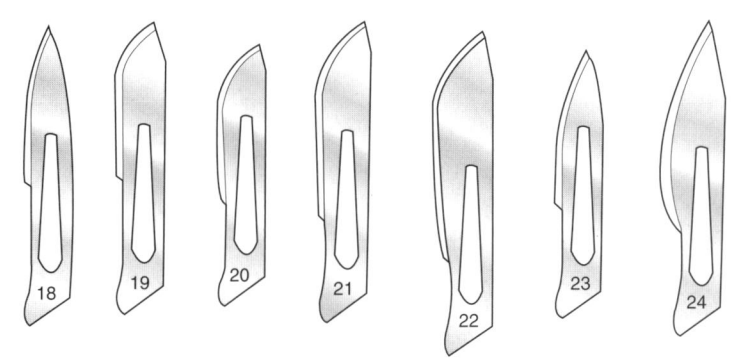

These larger blades are used for major incisions on a size 4 scalpel handle.

Fig. 2.3 *Large scalpel blades*

Scissors

Scissors are used to cut tissues during many parts of the dissection process and are produced in both sharp-pointed and blunt-ended varieties. The most commonly used in general surgery is blunt-ended. Other variations include straight, angled or curved blades, long or short bodies and light, medium or heavy gauge material. Each variant has its own particular use.

Scissors perform their cutting action by the two blades coming together in good apposition and so incising the tissue. This action will not occur if the blades don't meet. Blades may fail to meet if the scissors are damaged, or if they are too fine and so are forced apart by tissue bulk, or if the blade is incorrectly positioned by being held in the wrong hand. Tissue will then be torn and crushed by the 'chewing' action of the poorly meeting blades.

The curved variety of scissors has blades that follow the natural direction of a slightly flexed index finger and thereby act as an extension of it. It is this type that is used mostly in the dissection and division of tissues. In general, straight scissors are not recommended for cutting living tissue but are usually used for cutting sutures or dressings.

Scissors may also be used to dissect by inserting the blunt tips along a plane and spreading tissues apart by opening the blades, or by sliding the slightly opened blades along the line of tissue fibres (e.g. external oblique fascia). Longer or shorter models may be used for dissecting fine superficial structures or dissecting down in deep body cavities such as the pelvis. Sharp-pointed or angled scissors are often used for precision work such as opening small blood vessels or in fine dissection.

Most styles of scissors are designed for the right hand (unless specified otherwise) and a left-handed user has to force the blades together consciously for a smooth cutting action. They are also designed for use by a hand/forearm complex in the mid-prone position although, down a deep hole, the supinated position often gives the surgeon a better view of what is being cut.

To grip a pair of scissors properly the thumb is inserted into the upper ring and the ring finger inserted into the lower ring. The middle finger can then wrap round the shaft of the instrument, with the index finger positioned on the scissors joint or one of the shafts to steady the points. When using fine scissors, the wrist can be braced (in the same way as a scalpel) for improved accuracy of dissection. This practice is also useful when cutting sutures but the other hand is usually used for resting on (Fig. 2.4a, b).

When not being used the scissors may be swung on the ring finger to face back along the arm. They are held in place by the little finger thereby leaving the thumb, index and middle free to manipulate threads, instruments or other structures (Fig. 2.4c).

Basic Surgical Skills

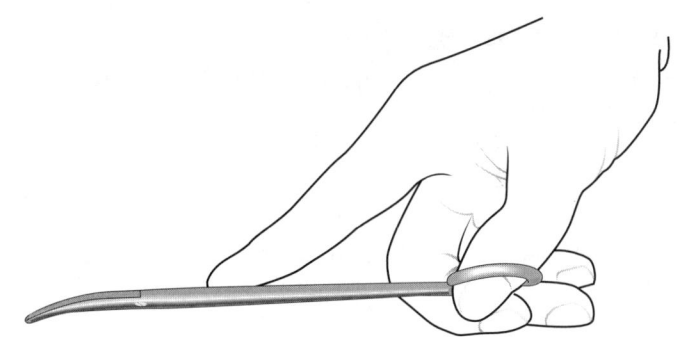

(a) Holding a pair of dissecting scissors

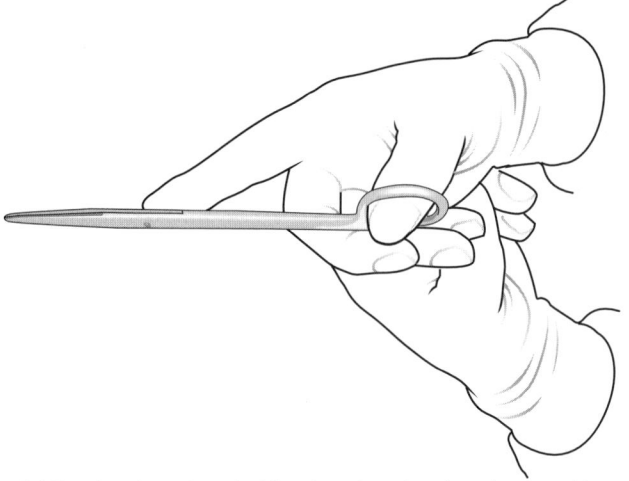

(b) Bracing the scissor-holding hand against the other hand for stability

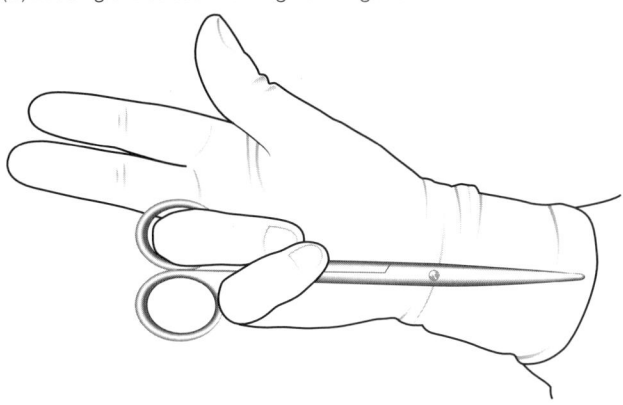

(c) 'Palming' scissors to free up the thumb, index and middle fingers for other functions

Fig. 2.4 *Holding scissors*

Dissecting scissors

The patterns of scissors shown in Figures 2.5 to 2.7 are used for dissecting tissues. They all have rounded points on both blades and are the most commonly used scissors in general surgery. Finer patterns, such as Metzenbaum's scissors, in long or short are one of the most commonly used scissors for basic dissection of soft tissues and intra-abdominal structures (e.g. adhesion division or bowel mobilisation). These invariably have curved blades. The heavier dissecting scissors such as Mayo scissors in the short variety, and Dubois or Golighers scissors in the long, also have curved blades and may be used in similar instances to those mentioned above. They come into their own, however, when cutting through thick fascia (e.g. rectus sheath or linea alba) or dissecting the mesorectum deep in the pelvis (Figs 2.5 to 2.7).

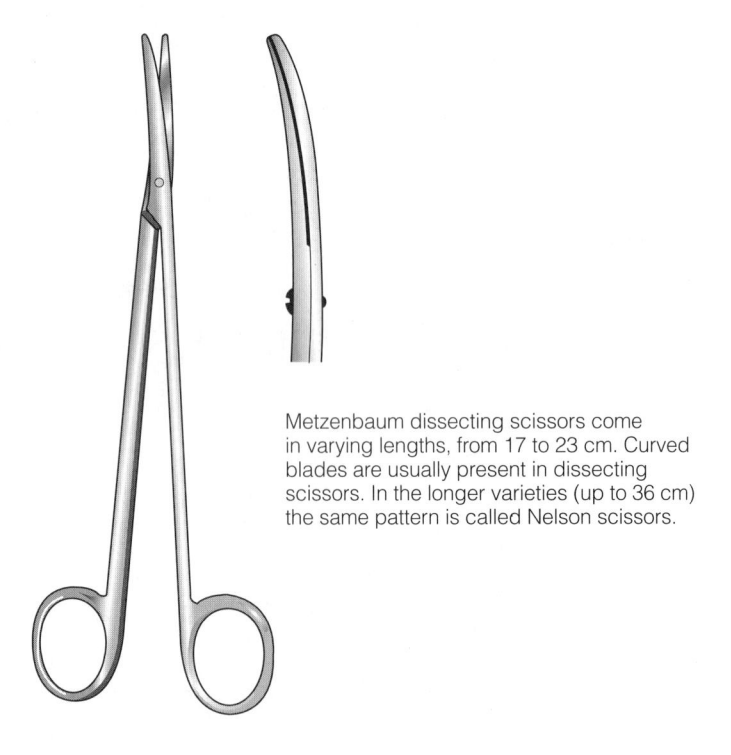

Metzenbaum dissecting scissors come in varying lengths, from 17 to 23 cm. Curved blades are usually present in dissecting scissors. In the longer varieties (up to 36 cm) the same pattern is called Nelson scissors.

Fig. 2.5 *Metzenbaum dissecting scissors*

Basic Surgical Skills

Some surgeons also use the curved Mayo scissors for tissue dissection.

They come in lengths from 14 to 23 cm.

(a) Curved Mayo scissors

(b) Straight Mayo scissors

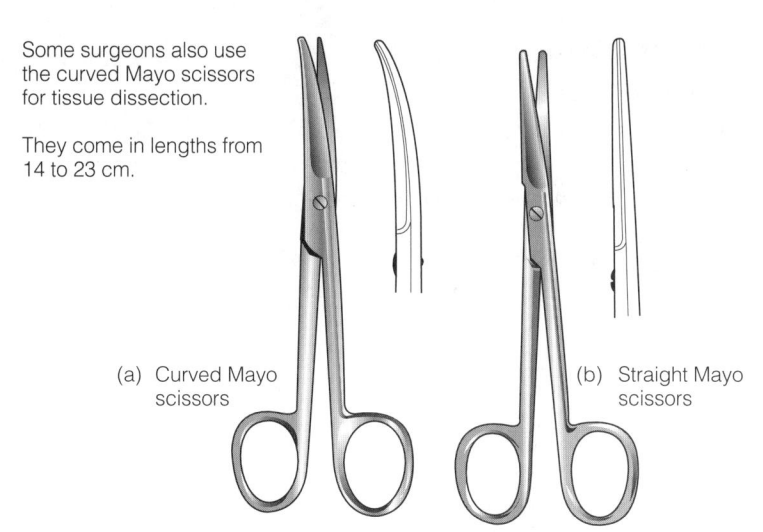

Fig. 2.6 *Mayo scissors*

These long heavy scissors (~ 30 cm) are now rarely used, even in pelvic surgery for which they were designed.

(a) Straight Dubois scissors

(b) Curved Dubois scissors

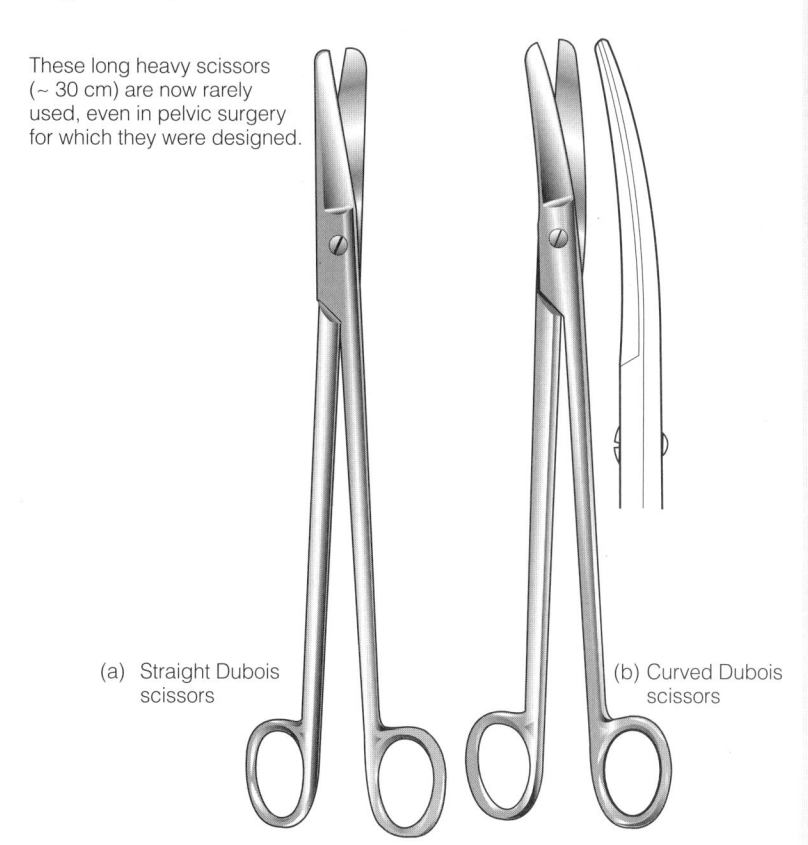

Fig. 2.7 *Dubois scissors*

Other scissors

Suture scissors
Ferguson's angled scissors are a commonly used pattern for this purpose (Fig. 2.8). Straight Mayo scissors, Nurses' scissors or any other straight-bladed scissor are also acceptable.

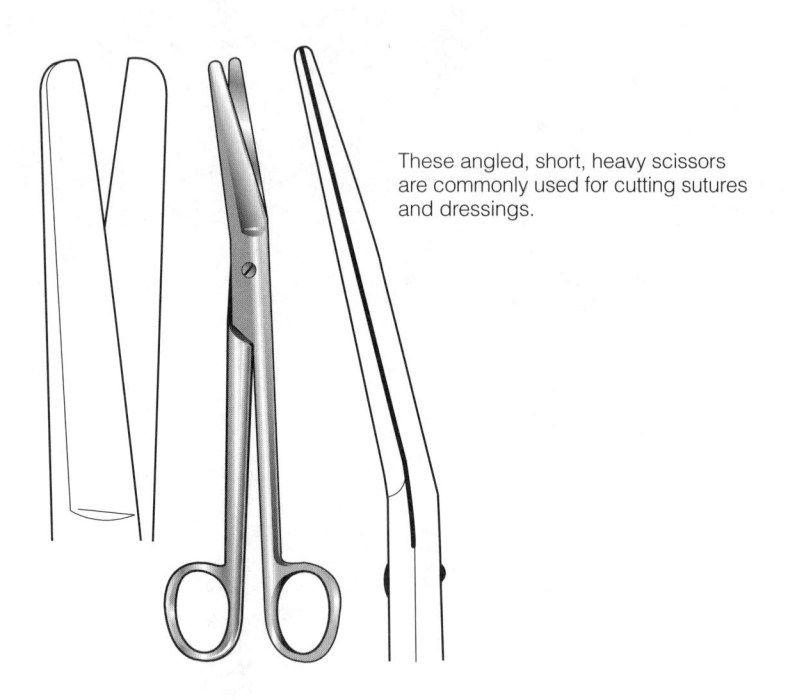

These angled, short, heavy scissors are commonly used for cutting sutures and dressings.

Fig. 2.8 *Ferguson scissors*

Dressing and general purpose scissors
Once again, straight-bladed Mayo scissors (Fig. 2.6) are popular for cutting dressings, stomal appliances, mesh or other materials but any heavy, straight-bladed, non-dissecting scissor is acceptable. Short styles such as Nurses' scissors are also designed for these tasks.

Vascular scissors
The most common vascular scissors are the Pott's angled scissors. This differs from the dissecting scissors in that it is angled (at anything up to 110°) and sharp-pointed to allow easier insertion into a vessel. There are various angles of blade depending on the situation. Pott's scissors are used exclusively to open blood vessels (Fig. 2.9).

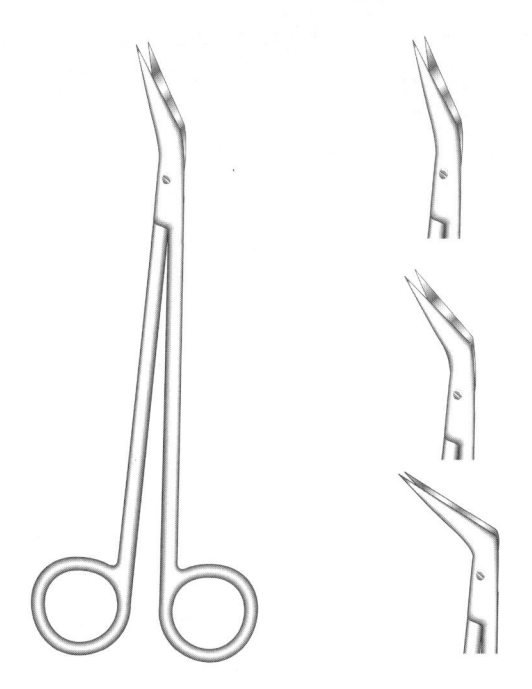

Pott's angled vascular scissors, with three differently angled blades. They are used for precision opening of blood vessels for surgery. The differently angled blades are used to reach vessels in deep or awkward positions.

Fig. 2.9 *Pott's scissors*

Other cutting instruments

While not used to dissect or incise in the same way as scalpels or scissors, there are several other cutting instruments that should be considered in this section.

Skin graft knife

This instrument has several variations in size, shape and complexity, ranging from a small knife that takes a single-sided razor blade through to a large electric skin graft harvester (dermatome). The function for which skin graft knives have been designed is the harvesting of flat sheets of uniform thickness skin containing the epidermis and part of the dermis. This leaves the lower dermis *in situ* (with its epidermal lined structures such as hair follicles) to heal by regenerating protective epidermis over its reduced thickness.

The illustrated instrument (Fig. 2.10) bears the eponymous title of the Watson modification of the Humby Knife. A long razor blade is inserted over the three lugs and the knobs on the end of the roller are used to adjust the aperture between the blade and the roller. This controls the thickness of skin harvested. The knife is held at an acute angle to the skin, which is first lubricated and then stretched tight and flattened by two small boards held by an assistant. The split skin is cut with a gentle to-and-fro sawing motion of the blade.

A smaller knife, the Silver knife, does the same job but holds only a single small blade and is useful for smaller grafts. An excellent dissertation on skin grafting can be found in McGregor's book *Fundamental Techniques of Plastic Surgery* (see reading list at end of chapter).

(a) Watson modification of the Humby Knife

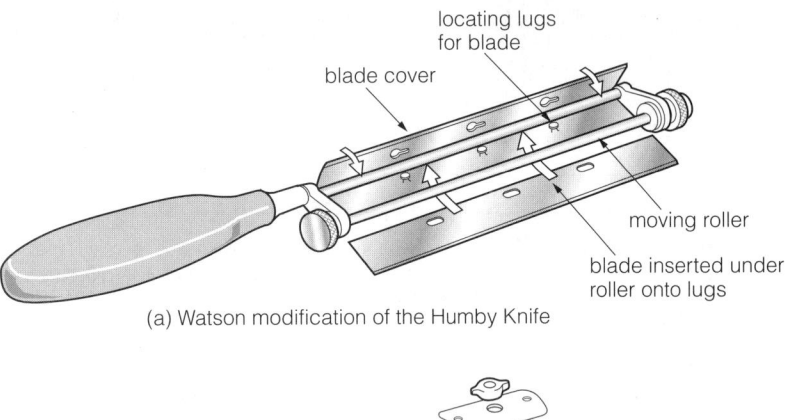

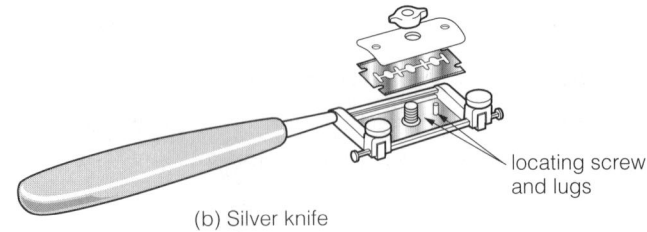

(b) Silver knife

Fig. 2.10 *Skin graft knives (left-handed versions shown)*

Bone cutters/nibblers

Traditionally used by orthopaedic surgeons, these instruments are also used in neurosurgery, thoracic surgery, vascular surgery, plastic surgery and any other specialty whose work involves the resection of bone. These instruments are shaped like scissors and have either heavy scissor-like blades (cutters) (Fig. 2.11) or a pair of scalloped cups (nibblers) (Fig. 2.12).

(a) Single-action bone cutters

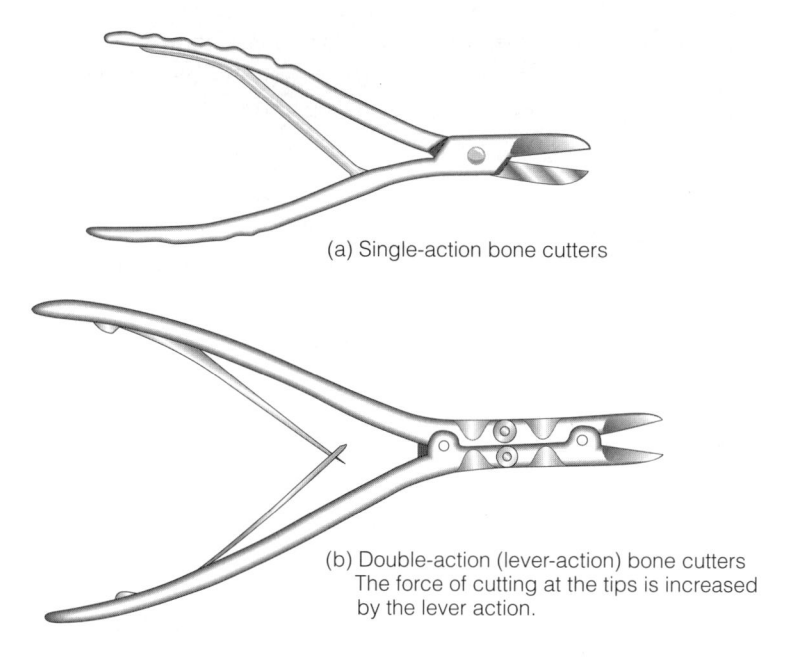

(b) Double-action (lever-action) bone cutters
The force of cutting at the tips is increased by the lever action.

Fig. 2.11 *Bone cutters*

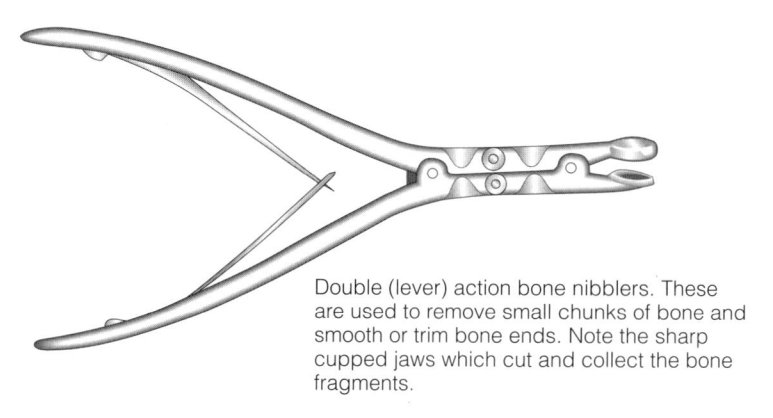

Double (lever) action bone nibblers. These are used to remove small chunks of bone and smooth or trim bone ends. Note the sharp cupped jaws which cut and collect the bone fragments.

Fig. 2.12 *Bone nibblers*

Periosteal elevator

Another instrument used in multiple specialties, the periosteal elevator lifts the periosteum (which contains osteocytes and their precursors) off bone prior to resecting it for either therapeutic or access reasons (e.g. ribs in thoracic surgery). At the conclusion of the case, replacement of the periosteum allows some bony regrowth in any space left without bone and aids bony healing. The periosteum first has to be incised by knife or diathermy and it is then literally pushed aside by the blunt, broad blade of the elevator (Fig. 2.13).

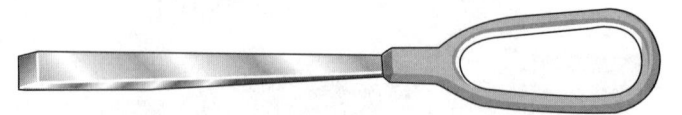

A periosteal elevator is used to lift the periosteum from bones before cutting them. The tip is sharp and angles down to a broad point.

Fig. 2.13 *Periosteal elevator*

Curette

This instrument, shaped essentially like a scoop, is used to clean out cavities by scraping away their contents. Abscesses, friable infected bone segments and the uterus are but a few of the situations in which this instrument is employed. The scoop-shaped head has a sharp edge that cuts away tissue as it scrapes against it. A curette is used by holding the handle in the palm of the hand, with the index finger extended along the instrument's shaft, then gently scraping the sharp edge of the scoop against the area containing the tissue to be removed (Fig. 2.14).

(a) Round-head curette

(b) Oval-head curette

The sharp edge of the scooped head cuts tissue as it scrapes the edges of the cavity.

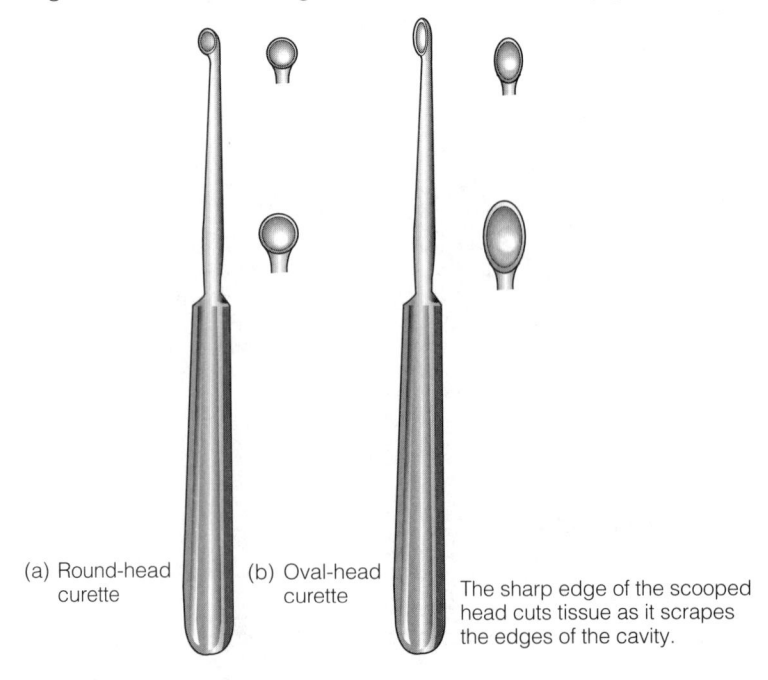

Fig. 2.14 *Curettes*

Grasping instruments

Forcep is the generic name given to any instrument that is used to grasp or hold. These may be hand-held (like tweezers) or in a scissor pattern, with or without a retaining ratchet. Forceps may be used to grasp tissues, needles, sutures or even other instruments. In this chapter grasping instruments are classified as:

1. tissue forceps
2. vascular forceps
3. needle-holding forceps
4. other grasping forceps

Tissue forceps

The basic purpose of tissue forceps is to grasp tissue, in a minimally traumatic manner, for stabilisation or retraction while performing another action such as suturing or dissecting. There are two basic designs of tissue forcep: hand-held patterns and scissor patterns.

The hand-held (or thumb) forcep comprises two blades of springy metal which are joined at the base, angle away from each other and then end at the same length with grooves or teeth on the tips. These tips meet and grasp if the two blades are squeezed together between the fingers and thumb.

To grip these instruments a 'chopstick' or 'penholding' grip is employed (Fig. 2.15a). The instrument is then balanced by resting it in the V between the thumb and index finger. Thumb forceps are generally used in the non-dominant hand to steady and display tissues, apply counter-pressure or provide tension against which to dissect. They may also be used for blunt dissection (with the tips held together) or for retracting

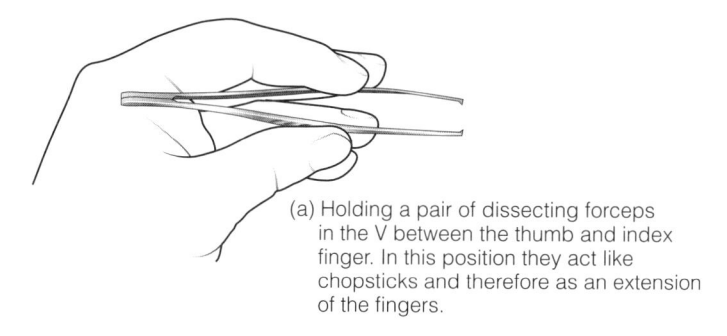

(a) Holding a pair of dissecting forceps in the V between the thumb and index finger. In this position they act like chopsticks and therefore as an extension of the fingers.

Fig. 2.15a *Holding hand-held forceps*

tissues in the same manner. Heavy and toothed variants are used for fascia and skin while finer non-toothed variants are used on viscera, vessels and other delicate structures.

When not in use these forceps may be 'palmed'—that is, wrapped into the palm and held firm by the ring and little fingers (Fig. 2.15b). Similar to palming scissors, this action leaves three fingers free to perform other tasks (e.g. tying).

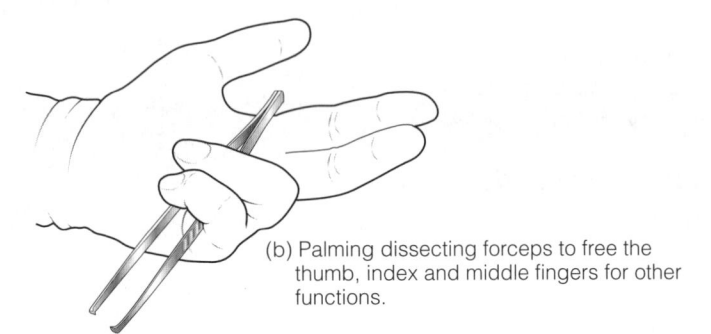

(b) Palming dissecting forceps to free the thumb, index and middle fingers for other functions.

Fig. 2.15b *Holding hand-held forceps*

The second type of tissue forcep has a ratcheted scissors shape and a pair of grasping tips on which grooves or teeth are present. When closed, the head may close flat to crush tissue or have a ring-like profile which allows tissue proximal to the tips to bulge between the jaws without compression or damage. A ratchet is used to lock the instrument in position while not being held. The instrument is gripped like a pair of scissors when applied. While grasping or retracting it may be held in the same way, or by the shaft below the finger rings (Fig. 2.16).

Holding a tissue forcep by the rings

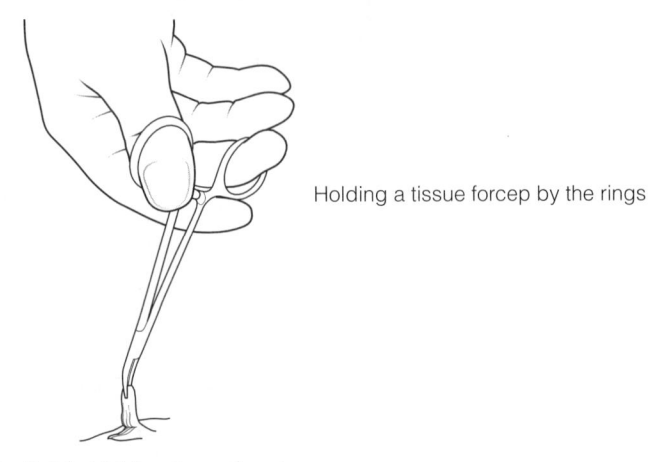

Fig. 2.16 *Holding tissue forceps*

Basic Surgical Skills

The main use for scissor-pattern ratcheted forceps is in stabilising or retracting tissues. They are especially useful when a strong grip is required for long periods of time, where a stay suture or hook may pull through or damage the tissue, if the tissues are too slippery to hold by hand or if the direction of retraction needs to be changed frequently. Heavy and toothed varieties are used on fascia and the finer, or atraumatic, tipped forceps are used on viscera.

Hand-held (thumb) forceps

These hand-held forceps, as described above, are for the manipulation of local soft tissues or viscera during the active phases of a procedure such as dissecting or suturing. They may be short, medium or long in size and their heads may be toothed or non-toothed depending on the tissue that is being handled.

Toothed forceps

Toothed hand-held forceps are commonly used for skin stabilisation (in the fine or medium patterns) or for fascia and muscle handling (in the heavy patterns) during the process of suturing. It is theorised that the presence of teeth on these forceps makes the grip required to hold the structures less forceful than if there were no teeth. This should mean that less trauma occurs to the tissues.

The number of teeth on each head (1 × 2 or 2 × 3, etc.) is dictated by the width of the head. The numbers refer to the number of teeth that interlock on the opposing heads (Fig. 2.17).

The numbers relate to the number of interlocking teeth on each head.

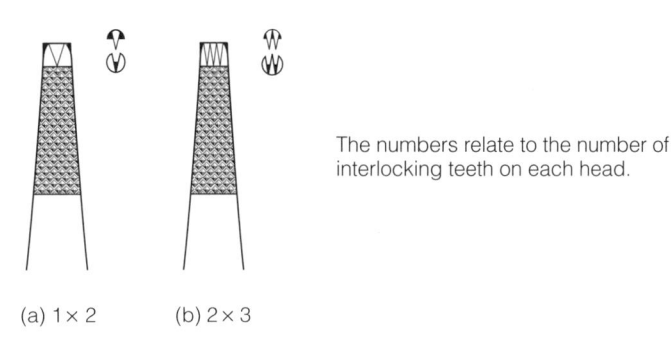

(a) 1 × 2   (b) 2 × 3

Fig. 2.17 *Toothed forcep heads*

Examples of toothed forceps are shown in Figure 2.18.

- **Small** (Fig 2.18a) Adson forceps (1 × 2 teeth) are fine-toothed forceps used mainly in plastic surgery or in the repair of minor

traumatic or surgical wounds. They are delicate and should only be used in areas of thin skin (i.e. not in the trunk or scalp, which are thick-skin areas).
- **Medium** (Fig. 2.18b)   Gillies forceps (1 × 2 teeth) are longer and slightly heavier than Adson forceps. They also have a post in the middle of one shaft that fits into a small hole in the opposing shaft to ensure tip alignment. They can be used for any type of skin.
- **Large** (Fig. 2.18c)   Lane's forceps (1 × 2 or 2 × 3) are used mainly for the grasping of bulky tissue during suturing (e.g. leg muscles in orthopaedic surgery or linea alba in abdominal closure). It is rare to use them on skin but they are excellent for heavy fascia, bone and cartilage.

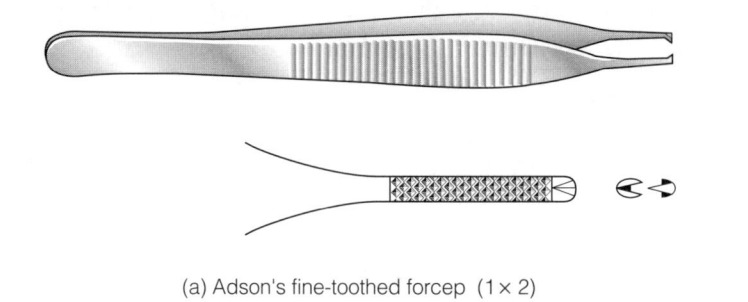

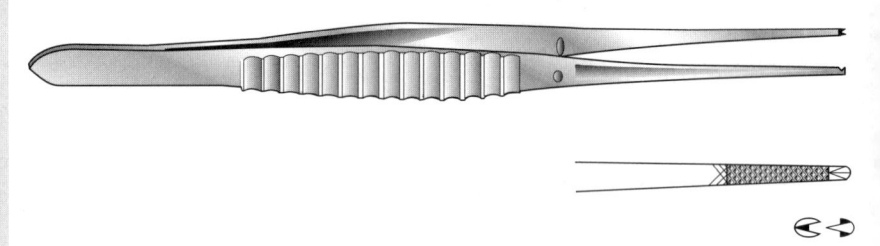

(a) Adson's fine-toothed forcep (1 × 2)

(b) Gillies medium toothed forcep (1 × 2)

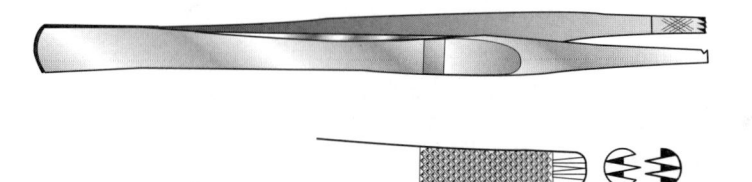

(c) Lane's heavy toothed forcep (2 × 3)

Fig. 2.18 *Toothed hand-held forceps*

Non-toothed forceps

There are two basic patterns of non-toothed forcep. The first genuinely has no teeth, only ridges or grooves on the surface of the tip. This type includes dressing forceps and McIndoe forceps (Fig. 2.19a). The second actually has interlocking longitudinal rows of teeth that are so small they are not easily discernible and are described as 'atraumatic' (Fig. 2.19b). One such pattern is known as a Debakey forcep after the American cardiovascular surgeon who designed it (Fig. 2.19c, d). There are several other variants on this theme that are not described here.

These forceps are used mostly for grasping viscera and serosal or adventitial surfaces, as the lack of teeth greatly lessens the likelihood of puncture. Debakey's forceps were designed as a vascular forcep but are commonly used for bowel and pulmonary work. Non-toothed forceps, of the grooved-head variety, are also used for manipulating packs and dressings both in theatre and on the wards.

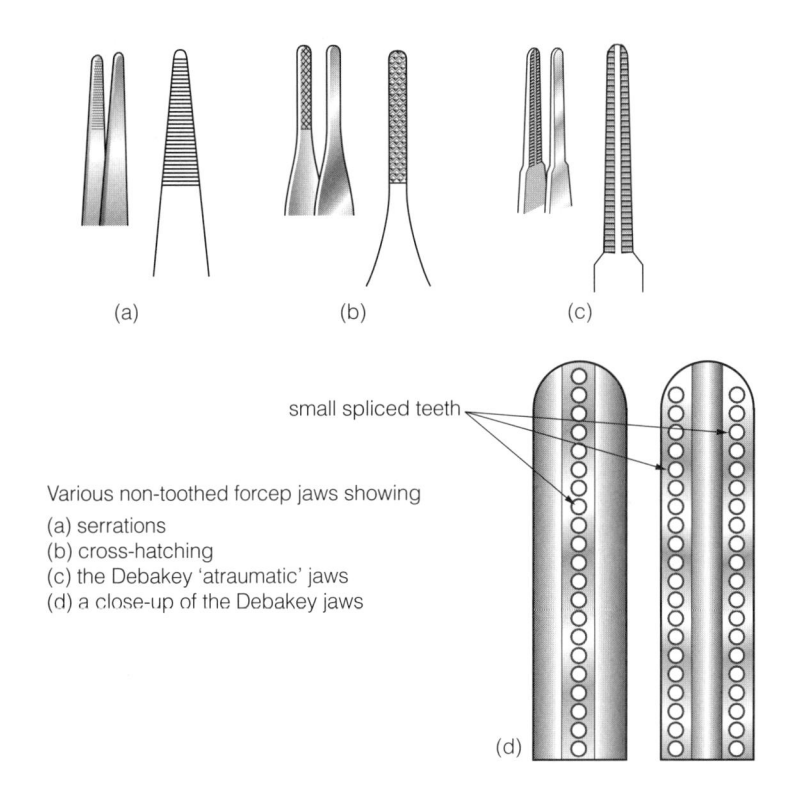

(a) (b) (c)

small spliced teeth

Various non-toothed forcep jaws showing
(a) serrations
(b) cross-hatching
(c) the Debakey 'atraumatic' jaws
(d) a close-up of the Debakey jaws

(d)

Fig. 2.19 *Non-toothed forcep jaws*

Examples of non-toothed forceps are shown in Figure 2.20.

- **Small/Short** These would usually be wound-dressing forceps (mostly on the ward) or small Debakey forceps for intricate vascular work.
- **Medium** Both types of non-toothed forcep come in this size but they are usually used for intraoperative visceral and vessel manipulation rather than for dressings.
- **Large/Long** Forceps in this size range are used predominantly in deep cavities (e.g. chest, pelvis for rectal surgery, or retroperitoneum for aortic surgery) where access for hand manipulation of tissues is severely limited. Once again both patterns exist, with the grooved variant serving the additional purpose of a 'packing' forcep, for the insertion of abdominal (gauze) packs to hold viscera out of the operative field.

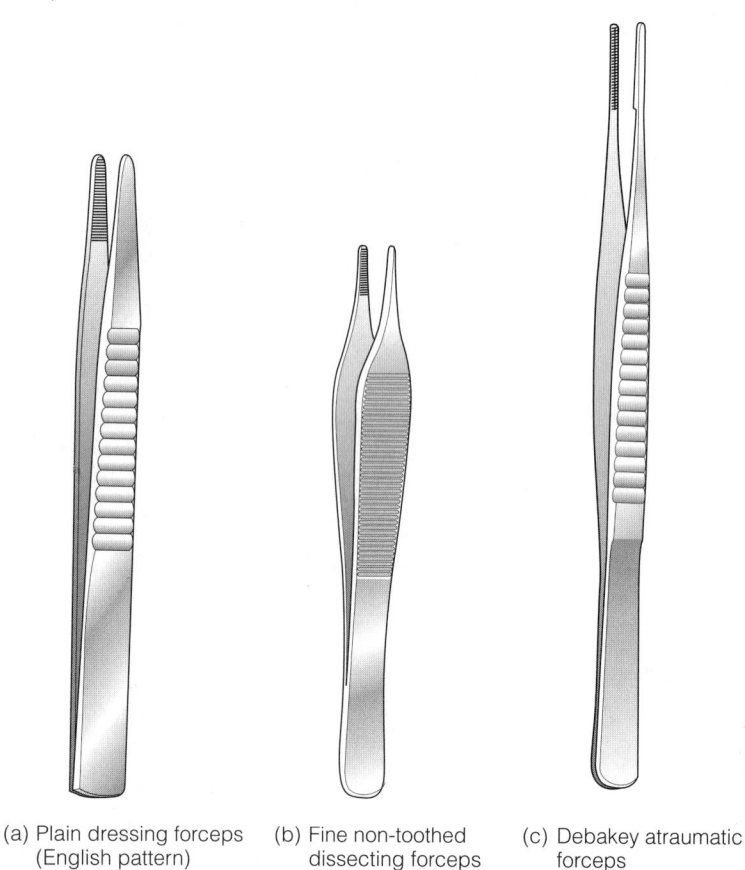

(a) Plain dressing forceps (English pattern)   (b) Fine non-toothed dissecting forceps   (c) Debakey atraumatic forceps

Fig. 2.20 *Non-toothed hand-held forceps*

Ratcheted (scissor-style) forceps

Ratcheted forceps can be used on any tissue depending on the instrument's 'heaviness', tip pattern (toothed or non-toothed) and head size. 'Heaviness' refers to both the gauge of metal from which the instrument is made and the force created at the instrument tips upon closure. The longer the distance from the joint to the tip of the jaws and the finer (or more flexible) the shafts of the instrument, the lesser the force that can be created. This concept is evident when comparing the force exerted at the tip of the long, fine bladed Babcock forcep compared with force of the short, heavy bladed Lane's forcep.

Toothed forceps

Toothed ratcheted forceps are used predominantly for grasping, stabilising and retracting structures. The actual tissue on which they are used depends on the size, strength and the tooth pattern on the instrument head, as detailed above.

- **Fine** Allis forceps are the commonest forcep in this category (Fig. 2.21a). As their head contains a row of short interlocking teeth and long fine bows (arms), they may be used for grasping bowel during suturing or for grasping dermis during subcutaneous dissection (e.g. in a mastectomy or thyroidectomy).
- **Heavy** Lane's, Kocher's and Rutherford-Morrison forceps are some common variants of this category (Fig. 2.21b, c). They have heavy, short bows, few long teeth and are commonly used to grasp heavy fascia or dermis.

Non-toothed forceps

As described above, the function of the non-toothed ratcheted forcep depends on the characteristics it possesses. In general, these forceps have much softer bows (arms) for lower pressure on the head when closed and are therefore commonly used on viscera. Use on harder or thicker tissues inevitably leads to slippage and this may be dangerous at the vital point of a procedure.

- **Fine** Babcock forceps have a rounded head and grooved tips (Fig. 2.22a). They are commonly used for grasping bowel or other viscera because of their softness. They cannot be used for heavy or bulky tissue as they inevitably slip.
- **Heavy** Duvall forceps have a large triangular head with grooves or tiny teeth (Fig. 2.22b). Again their grip is quite soft but as they have a large gripping area, bulky viscera such as lung and stomach are well held by them.

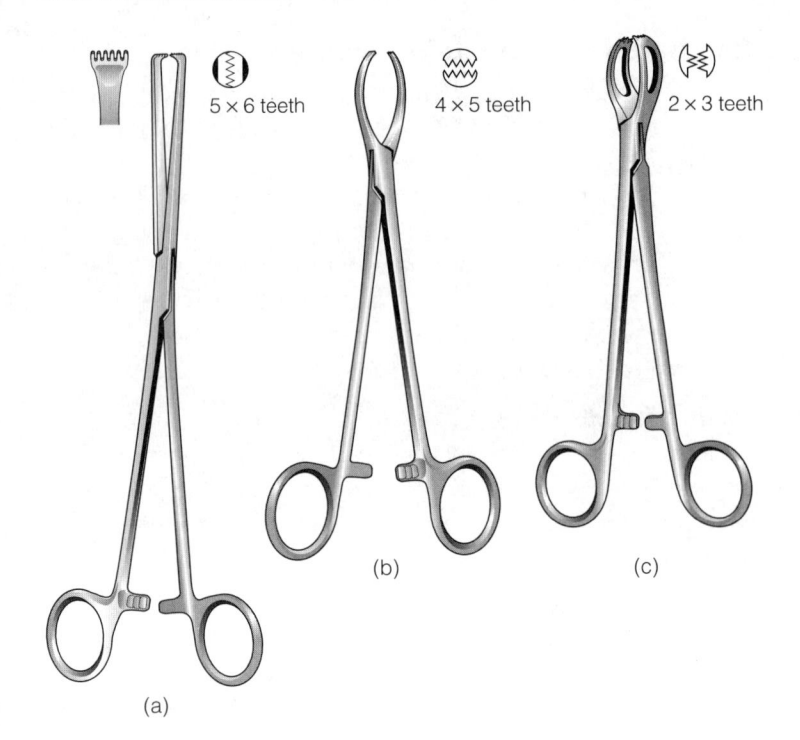

(a) Allis forcep showing long, fine arms and a 5×6 tooth configuration
(b) Rutherford-Morrison forcep showing shorter, stronger arms and a 4×5 tooth configuration
(c) Lane's forcep showing very short, heavy arms and a 2×3 tooth configuration

Fig. 2.21 *Toothed ratcheted forceps*

Vascular forceps

Vascular forceps can be categorised generically into two broad groups—crushing and non-crushing. As with tissue-holding forceps the gauge of material, length of shafts and type of tips will dictate their function.

In broad terms the crushing, or haemostatic, type are used to grip vessels, and sometimes some of the tissue surrounding them, with the aim of controlling bleeding from these sites and presenting them for ligation. They are generally referred to as artery forceps and are not a true vascular clamp. They can also function as tissue-holding forceps similar to those described in the previous section (Fig. 2.23).

Basic Surgical Skills

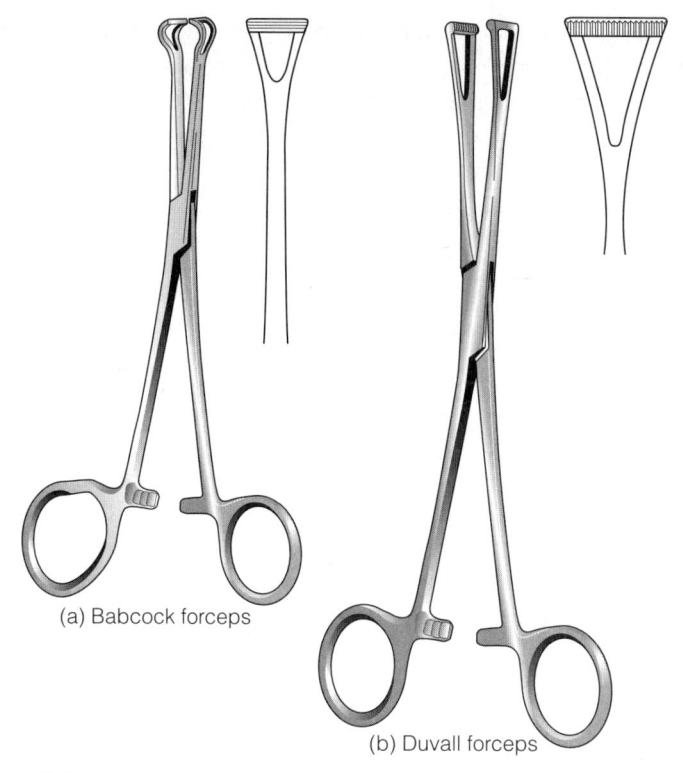

(a) Babcock forceps

(b) Duvall forceps

Fig. 2.22 *Non-toothed ratcheted forceps*

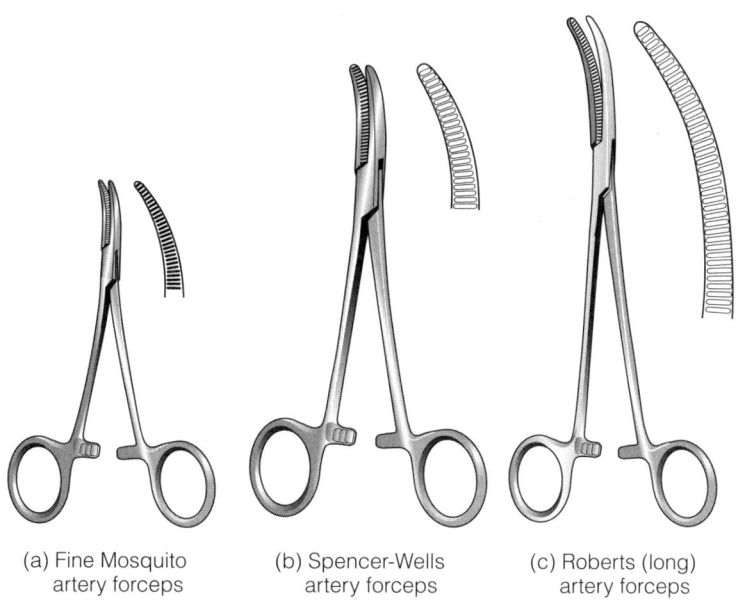

(a) Fine Mosquito artery forceps

(b) Spencer-Wells artery forceps

(c) Roberts (long) artery forceps

Fig. 2.23 *Haemostatic vascular (artery) forceps*

Non-crushing vascular clamps, on the other hand, are used for the temporary occlusion of a vessel while some form of surgical procedure is being performed upon it (e.g. endarterectomy or arterial bypass). They exert a pressure at the tips which is adequate for preventing blood flow through the occluded vessel, but not so great as to damage the vessel to any major extent. These instruments are regarded as true vascular clamps (Fig. 2.24).

(a) Angled Debakey vascular clamp

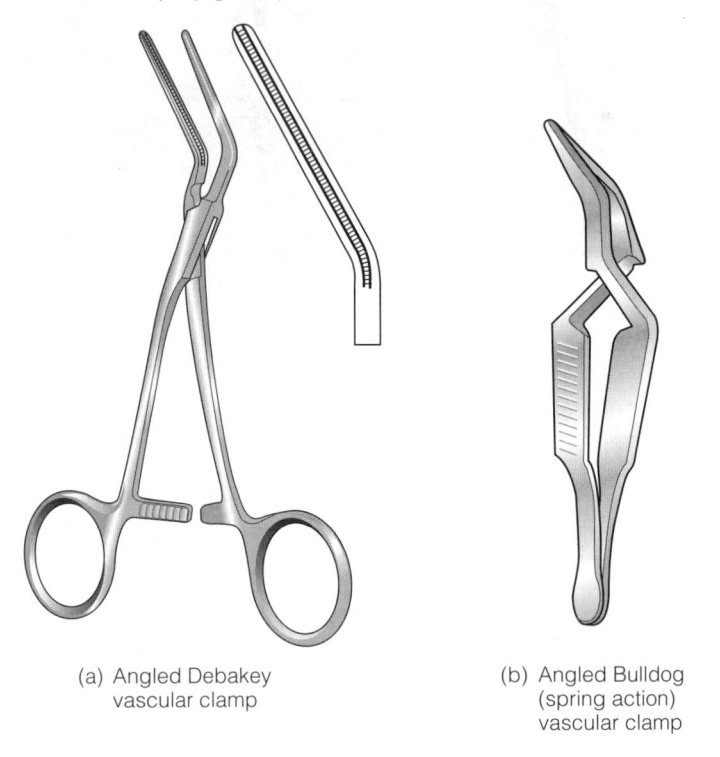

(b) Angled Bulldog (spring action) vascular clamp

Fig. 2.24 *Non-crushing vascular clamps*

To remove a vascular forcep the fingers may be reinserted into the rings and the reverse of application carried out. If the angle is wrong for this, the thumb is applied to the proximal ring of the forceps and the next two fingers to the distal ring. These fingers can then apply pressure to disengage the ratchet and the forcep can be removed in one smooth action.

Haemostatic artery forceps

Artery forceps are shaped like scissors with either straight or curved jaws of varying stiffness (Fig. 2.23). These instruments are applied while being held like scissors. The tips oppose first in closing and the jaws come together, crushing all tissue between them. Care must be taken to include only the vessel and minimal extra tissue. If excessive tissue is grasped the tie may only be secured on this and the vessel may retract and bleed. Adjacent (often important) structures should also be carefully avoided.

When an artery forceps is applied across a vessel the tips should protrude just beyond the grasped tissue so that a ligature can be slipped below the same. If this does not occur, a second pair that does protrude must be applied below the first forcep. The ratchet must be clicked enough to ensure crushing of the tissues and a secure grip. Over-tightening, however, may cut through thick or oedematous tissue and cause the forceps to spring apart in an uncontrolled fashion when released.

Non-toothed forceps

Usually just called artery forceps, these instruments have various eponymous names based on their length, heaviness, variations in shape and local custom. Short and fine variants are often known as Mosquito forceps, the medium style in both may be called Spencer-Wells forceps or Halsted forceps, depending on their shape, and the longer and heavier style are commonly known as Roberts forceps. There are many other combinations, such as a long and fine forcep, that will not be dealt with here.

In general, the curved variety of artery forcep is used on tissues and vessels, and the straight form used to hold sutures. When applied, the traditional method is to have the concavities of the head facing into the wound. This makes slipping a ligature beneath the blades much easier as the tips then also face into the wound (Fig. 2.25).

Toothed forceps

Toothed artery forceps come in small and large varieties and the eponymous name for all sizes is Kocher's forceps (Fig. 2.26). They are generally heavier than the non-toothed forcep and the tooth aids both in gripping tissue and preventing tissue from squeezing out the open end of the jaws. They are excellent for clamping particularly bulky tissues before division (e.g. uterine or ovarian vessels) or for substitution as a crushing bowel clamp.

Basic Surgical Skills

vessel
artery forcep

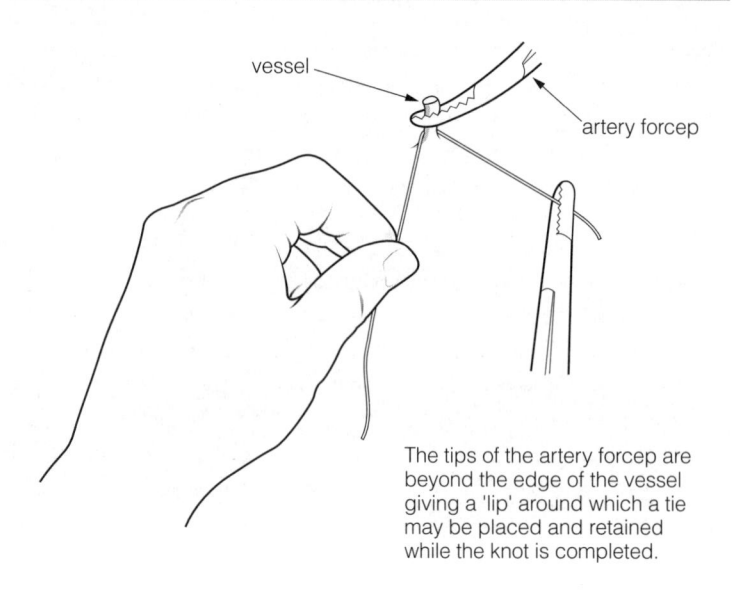

The tips of the artery forcep are beyond the edge of the vessel giving a 'lip' around which a tie may be placed and retained while the knot is completed.

Fig. 2.25 *Positioning an artery forcep on a vessel*

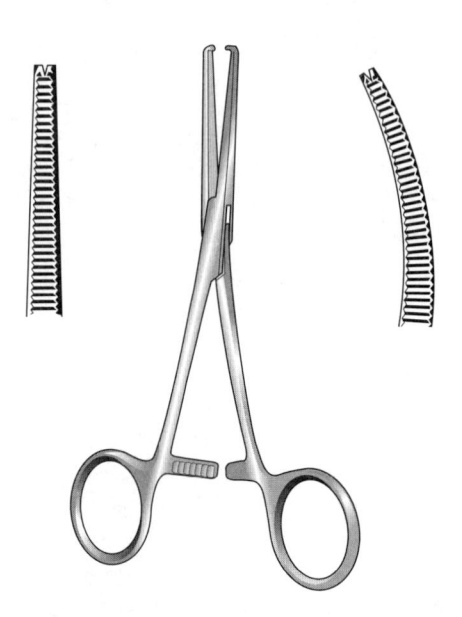

Fig. 2.26 *Kocher's forceps*

Basic Surgical Skills

Vascular clamps (non-crushing)

True vascular clamps are made in a ratcheted scissor style and in a 'spring', or bulldog, style that works like a clothes peg (Fig. 2.24). These instruments are purpose-designed to temporarily prevent the flow of blood through a vessel while it is being operated upon. Importantly, their design incorporates features which prevent crushing of the tissues and subsequent intimal damage (and hence a risk of intravascular thrombosis).

Vascular clamps have a pattern of atraumatic serrations along their jaw, as opposed to formal teeth. Different angles, curves and jaw-grip patterns are based on the type of vessel they will be used on and on whether all, or only some, of the vessel lumen requires occlusion. Some vascular clamps even have gel-filled cushions on the grasping side of the jaw to help prevent trauma. They are also produced in different lengths and weights (fine, medium and heavy varieties) for different vessel types (Fig. 2.27).

The scissor style is used in the same way as an artery forcep while the clothes-peg style rests in the closed position and requires squeezing to open the jaws. The blades of these forceps come together flatly, as opposed to the tip-first closure of an artery forcep. The clothes-peg style forcep has a set occlusion pressure whereas the scissor style is ratcheted and should only be tightened enough to occlude, **not damage**, the vessels it is applied to. When applied, neither type must include any extra tissue as this will reduce their effectiveness. The tips of each should only just protrude beyond the vessel so as not to present an obstacle that must be avoided.

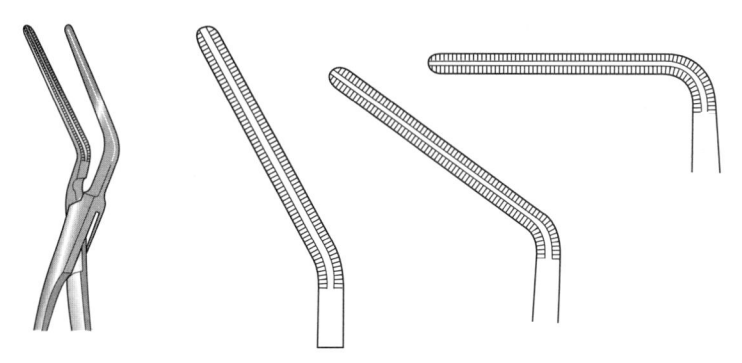

(a) A variety of angled blades for the Debakey angled vascular clamp

Fig. 2.27a *Vascular clamp jaw patterns*

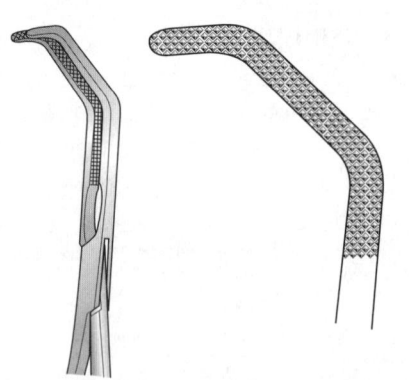

(b) The Satinsky vascular clamp, used to occlude part of the lumen of a vessel for operation

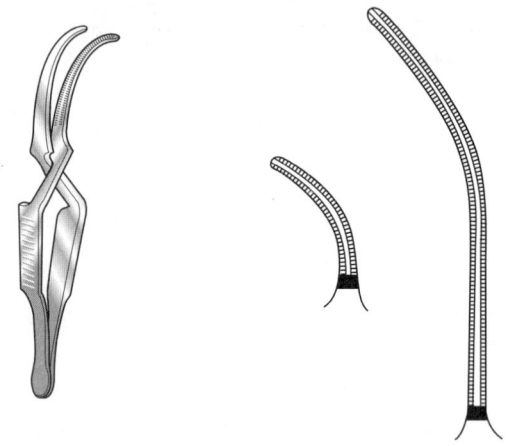

(c) Long and short blades for the curved Bulldog vascular clamp

Fig. 2.27b, c *Vascular clamp jaw patterns*

Needle-holding forceps

Needle-holding forceps are used to insert (or drive) a needle, attached to a suture thread, through tissues. These forceps may have a locking ratchet or may be non-locking. If there is a ratchet the forcep may be constructed in a classic scissor pattern or have long curved shafts with no finger rings (Fig. 2.28).

The jaws of a needle holder are required to provide a strong grip on the needle. To this end, they are usually short compared with the length of the shafts, thus ensuring a strong grip at the tips. The jaws are usually lined with cross-hatching or serrated tungsten carbide inserts (Fig. 2.29).

Basic Surgical Skills

(a) Mayo-Hegar needle-holding forcep

(b) Ryder vascular needle-holding forcep

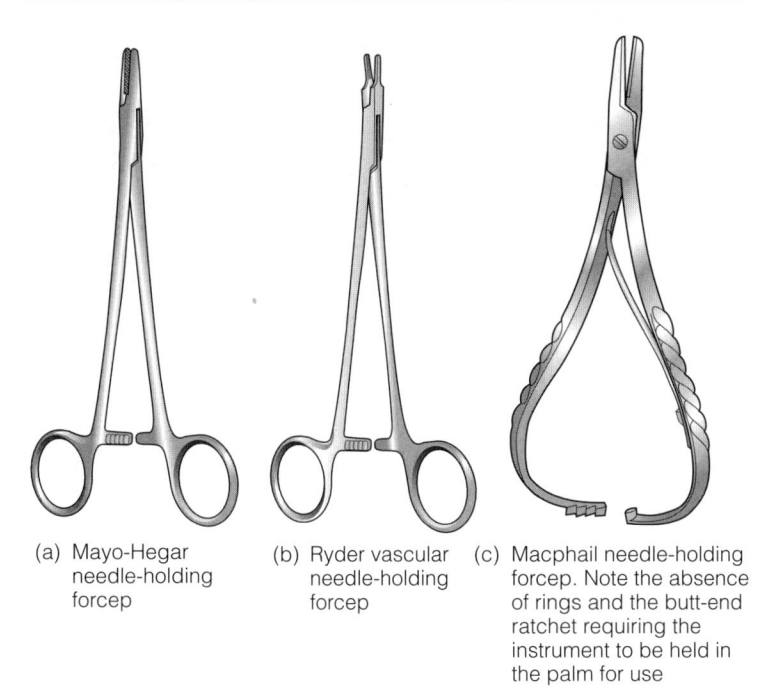

(c) Macphail needle-holding forcep. Note the absence of rings and the butt-end ratchet requiring the instrument to be held in the palm for use

Fig. 2.28 *Ratcheted needle-holding forceps*

(a) Cross-hatched and grooved Mayo-Hegar jaws

front   side

(b) Tungsten carbide cross-hatched insert for the Mayo-Hegar needle holder (front and side views)

(c) Fine Ryder vascular needle holder jaws

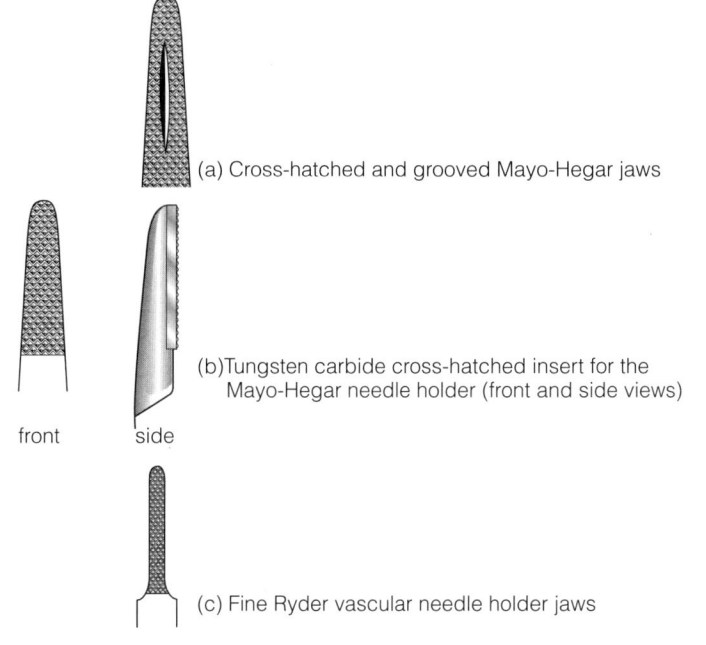

Fig. 2.29 *Needle holder jaws*

Surgical instruments and their uses

Needle-holding forceps need to be held in a particular way to be effective. You will learn in greater detail later that a needle is usually inserted by either pronation or supination of the forearm. This generally means that the hand and wrist are locked in position during the process of insertion. The instrument must be held, therefore, with its long axis in the line of the forearm. To achieve this the wrist is slightly ulnar deviated, the thumb placed in or on the upper finger ring of the needle holder, the index finger placed on the joint and the other three fingers curled around the lower finger ring. The 4th finger may be placed in the lower finger ring if this is more comfortable (Fig. 2.30a). If correctly held, the tip of the forceps should remain at the same point in space and merely rotate along the long axis of the instrument and forearm when the arm is pronated and supinated. If the tip itself describes an arc of movement, the alignment is not quite correct.

The alternative position is to place the needle holder in the palm of the hand with the upper ring against the thenar eminence, the length of the holder along the index finger and the other three fingers wrapped around the lower finger ring (Fig. 2.30b).

Non-ratcheted needle holders often have the upper shaft shorter than the lower. This allows the long axis of the instrument and the forearm to match with the thumb and finger inserted into the finger holes and the wrist not having to be ulnar deviated.

Once again, all these forceps may be palmed by swinging them back into the palm of the hand with the 4th finger inserted through the lower finger ring, similar to the position used for scissors (Fig. 2.4c). An alternative method involves placing the instrument flat in the palm and wrapping the ring and little fingers around it, similar to the position for hand-held forceps (Fig. 2.15b). These techniques should only be used if the needle is not in the holder or is securely protected by reversing it to point into the joint of the needle holder (Fig. 2.31). Palming is especially useful during suturing as it means that the needle-holding forcep does not have to be put down and then retrieved during hand tying.

The needle holder may also be used to tie sutures, especially in the subcutaneous tissue or skin.

Locking needle-holding forceps

The commonest pattern of needle holder in general surgical use is the Mayo-Hegar variety. This is a ratcheted scissor pattern that has a short, grooved head with a central pit in the blade. These can be made in

Basic Surgical Skills

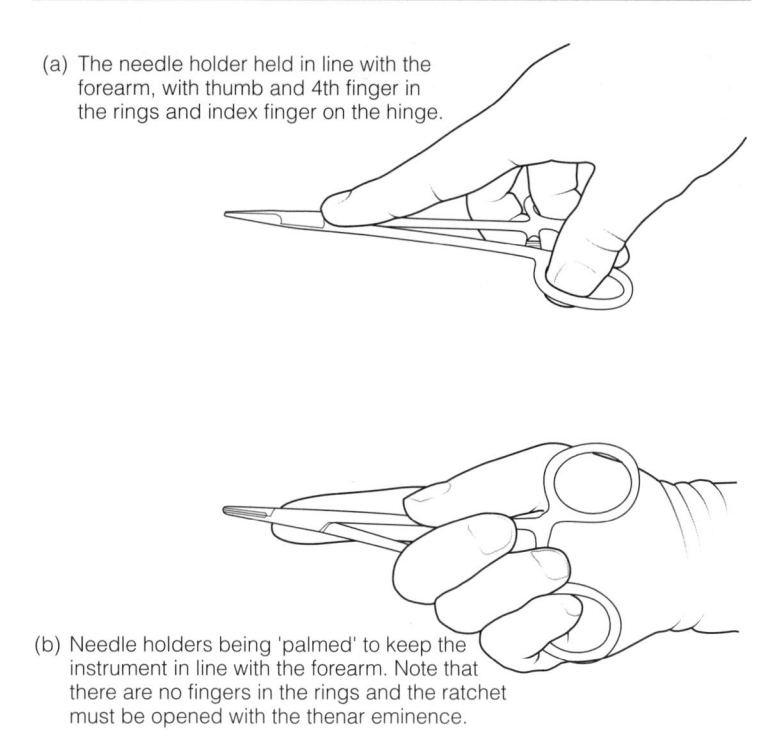

(a) The needle holder held in line with the forearm, with thumb and 4th finger in the rings and index finger on the hinge.

(b) Needle holders being 'palmed' to keep the instrument in line with the forearm. Note that there are no fingers in the rings and the ratchet must be opened with the thenar eminence.

Fig. 2.30 *Two methods of holding a needle holder*

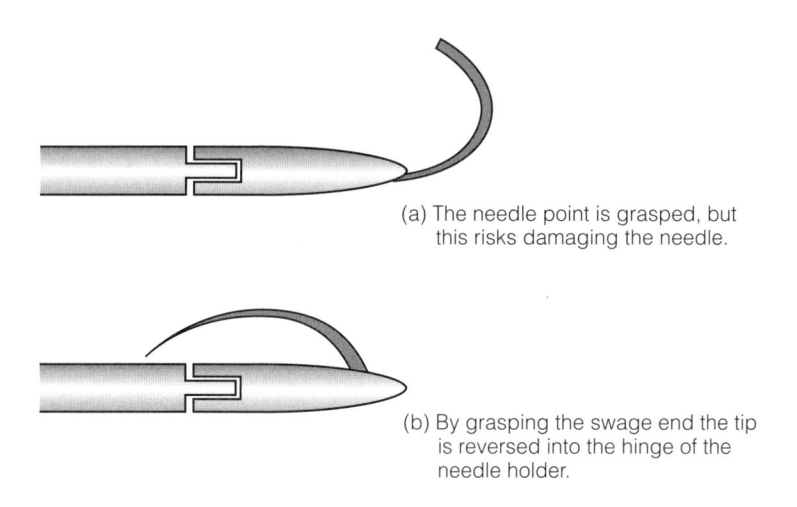

(a) The needle point is grasped, but this risks damaging the needle.

(b) By grasping the swage end the tip is reversed into the hinge of the needle holder.

Fig. 2.31 *Two methods of protecting the point of a needle when passing a needle-holding forcep*

virtually any length. Finer needle holders for vascular or plastic surgical work include the Ryder, Olsen-Hegar, Gillies and Crile-Wood patterns. These come in short and long varieties. In general, the length of the needle holder should be such that the hand using it is out of the operative field and does not obstruct the operator's view. This, of course, must be tempered by the length being reasonable from a control point of view.

Non-locking needle-holding forceps

The most common non-locking needle holder is the Gillies pattern. It has a shorter upper shaft and large thumb ring angled away from the axis of the instrument. A pair of scissors is incorporated in the blades and the jaws are slightly curved. They are used almost exclusively by plastic surgeons.

The Gillies needle holder is significantly more difficult to use than a conventional, ratcheted needle holder, as constant pressure needs to be applied to the blades in order to retain a grip on the needle. In its favour the size, shape and features of this needle holder allow for easy handling and tying (there is no ratchet) and cutting of one's own sutures, thereby improving ergonomics (Fig. 2.32).

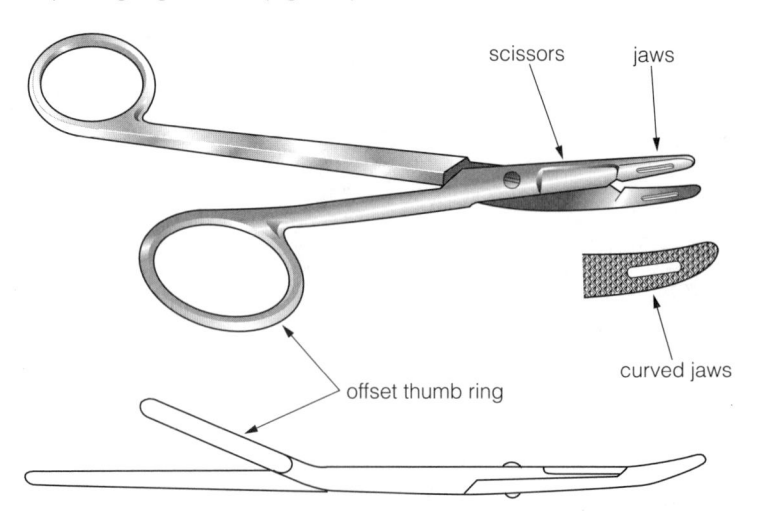

Fig. 2.32 *Gillies needle holder*

Other types of forcep

A variety of specialised forceps fall into the general categories discussed above but they rate a mention on an individual basis because of their frequent use and special functions.

Bowel clamps

When dealing with bowel there are situations where it is desirable to occlude the lumen without damaging the bowel, or to crush the bowel to ensure a watertight seal before it is divided. Specialised non-crushing and crushing clamps have been designed for these purposes. There are multiple patterns of both and many will not be dealt with here.

Non-crushing bowel clamps

Doyen non-crushing bowel clamps are scissor-pattern, ratcheted clamps with a pair of long and very flexible blades. These blades are significantly longer than the handles above the instrument's joint, thereby ensuring lower pressures at the tip. The flexibility and width of the blades further lessen the pressure. Non-crushing bowel clamps may be either straight or curved and the blades usually have longitudinal grooves and micro-teeth, similar to Debakey forceps. The tips meet first and the long blades then come gently together to occlude the lumen of the bowel without interrupting the blood supply. When applying these clamps, care must be taken not to crush the mesentery between the tips as this may cause vessel damage and ischaemia (Fig. 2.33).

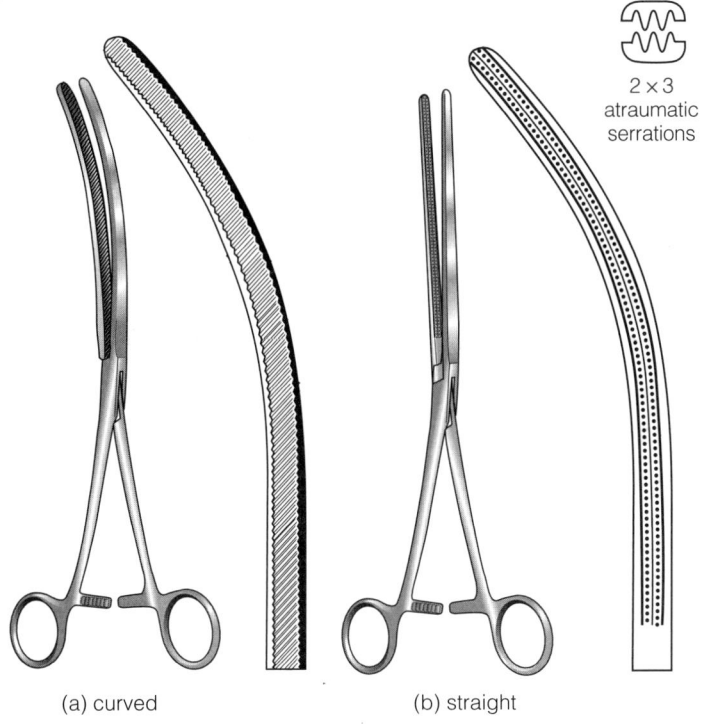

2 × 3 atraumatic serrations

(a) curved (b) straight

Doyen soft bowel clamps with different jaw patterns: Debakey and cross-hatched

Fig. 2.33 *Non-crushing bowel clamps*

Crushing bowel clamps

Lang-Stevenson crushing bowel clamps are just one variety of these. Once again this is a ratcheted scissor-pattern clamp with longitudinally grooved blades that are strong and virtually rigid (Fig. 2.34). The bowel is crushed between the jaws before it is divided at the edge of the instrument. In general, crushing bowel clamps are used on the specimen side of the bowel with non-crushing clamps placed on the side to be retained and anastomosed. Other similar clamps include Parker-Kerr clamps, Kocher's forceps and various angled rectal clamps.

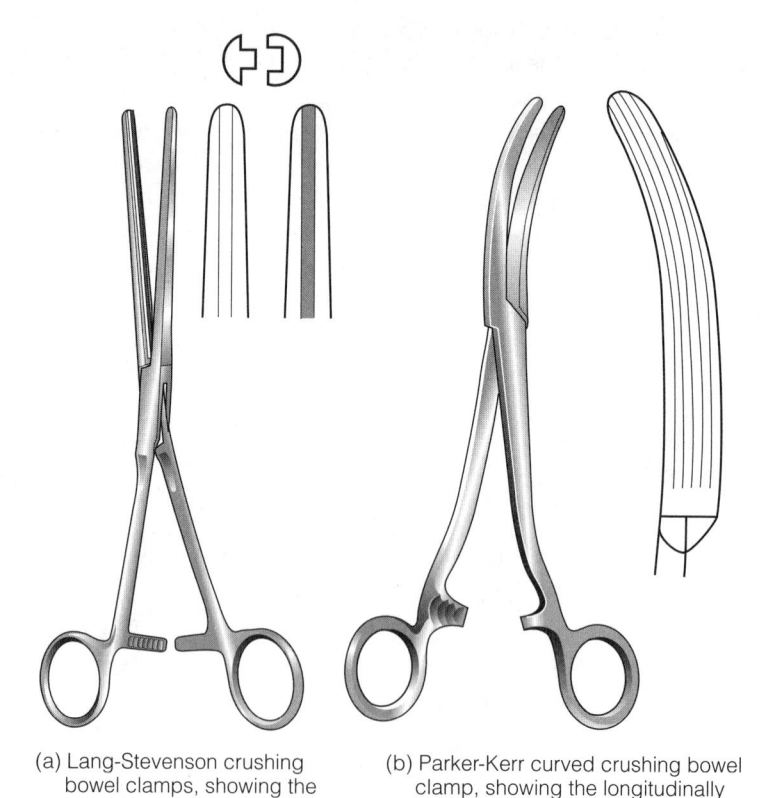

(a) Lang-Stevenson crushing bowel clamps, showing the grooved keyed blades

(b) Parker-Kerr curved crushing bowel clamp, showing the longitudinally ridged blades

Fig. 2.34 *Crushing bowel clamps*

Gall-bladder forceps

While many different forceps may be used to hold the gall bladder during an open procedure, including Rampley's sponge-holding forceps (Fig. 2.37), the most common is the Moynihan forcep. This is a scissor-pattern, ratcheted, non-toothed, curved-blade forcep. It grips well due to its rigidity and the cross-hatching on the blades. It is also sometimes used as a substitute for a long, heavy artery forcep (Fig. 2.35).

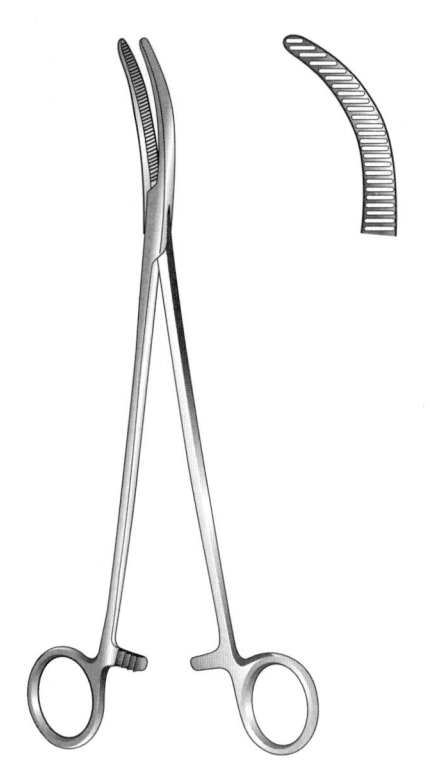

Fig. 2.35 *Moynihan gall-bladder forceps*

Right-angled forceps

This generic name applies to any scissor-pattern, ratcheted forcep in which the jaws undergo a (virtually) 90° bend during their course. These instruments come in fine and heavy variants and are very useful for passing sutures, or slings, around or under structures deep in a wound. They can also be used to grasp blood vessels in a deep cavity. In this situation the right-angled jaw will clamp across the vessel whereas a long (straight or curved) artery forcep would grasp the vessel end-on, making for a much more difficult tie. Common patterns include Lahey forceps and the finer Mixter forceps (Fig. 2.36).

(a) Lahey angled forceps (b) Mixter right-angled forceps

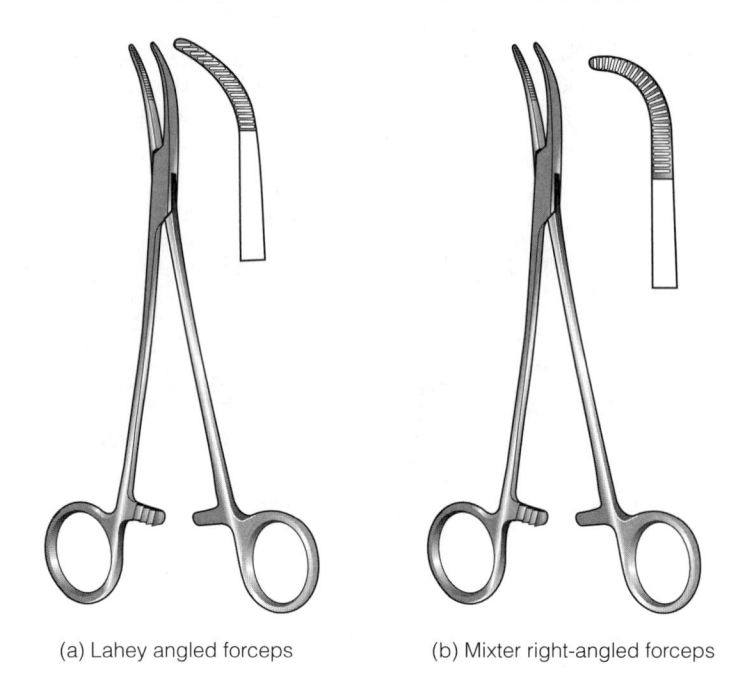

Fig. 2.36 *Right-angled forceps*

Sponge-holding forceps

The Rampley sponge-holding forcep is another long, scissor-pattern, ratcheted forcep. It is used to hold the swabs with which the skin is prepared preoperatively and to hold 'Raytec' gauzes for blotting tissues dry during dissection. It may also be used as a tissue forcep for the gall bladder or lung (Fig. 2.37).

Retracting instruments

Retractors are an essential tool for the display of deep tissues by the assistant during an operation. They may be held by hand, or they may be a self-retaining pattern that locks into position with a spring, ratchet or screw mechanism.

The essential principle of retraction is the placement of a blade in front of tissue that would otherwise reduce visibility in the operative field. The blade may be used passively to prevent tissue falling into the wound or for active (and sometimes necessarily forceful) retraction of tissues out of the wound. Great care must be taken in this latter situation that damage is not caused to the structures being retracted. This is the art of retraction.

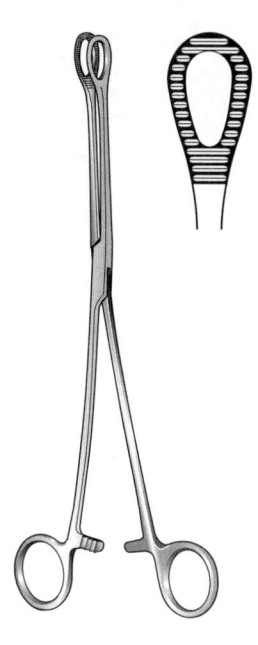

Fig. 2.37 *Rampley's sponge-holding forceps*

Hand-held retractors

These are held in position by one of the assistants to displace or prevent ingress of tissues into the operative field. If properly handled they are minimally traumatic as pressure on the underlying structures can be varied as the need for exposure alters. All retractors have a 'blade' of some description set at approximately right angles to a long, sometimes thin, handle. Exposure is achieved by a combination of judicious placement, careful pull and 'toe in' rotation of the blade. 'Toe in' movement is achieved by lifting the retractor handle away from the skin surface and keeping the bend of the retractor fixed, thus angling the toe of the retractor further into the patient (Fig. 2.38).

There are many sizes and patterns of retractor for specific retraction tasks and we deal with a few of the common ones in this section.

Small hand-held retractors
Toothed small hand-held retractors
The common small, toothed retractors include the skin hook, the cats-paw retractor and the rake retractor. These instruments are used predominantly for the retraction of skin edges during minor skin surgery. They grip well because all have pointed teeth (similar to a curved fork)

Basic Surgical Skills

and are also very secure. The cats-paw retractor also has a small right-angled blade at the opposite end from the points (Fig. 2.39).

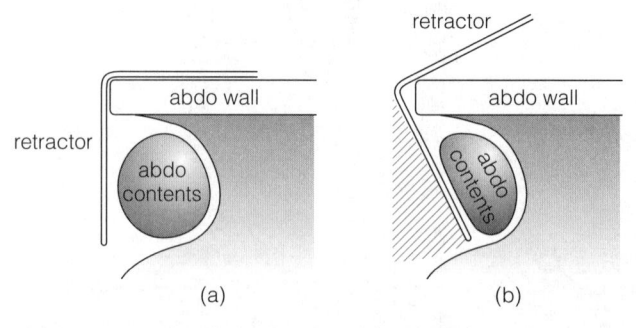

As the retractor handle is lifted from (a) to (b) the toe of the retractor rotates 'into' the patient. This increases the exposure (as shown by the hatched area) but puts the underlying structures at risk from pressure exerted by the retractor.

Fig. 2.38 *'Toe-in' as applied to retractors*

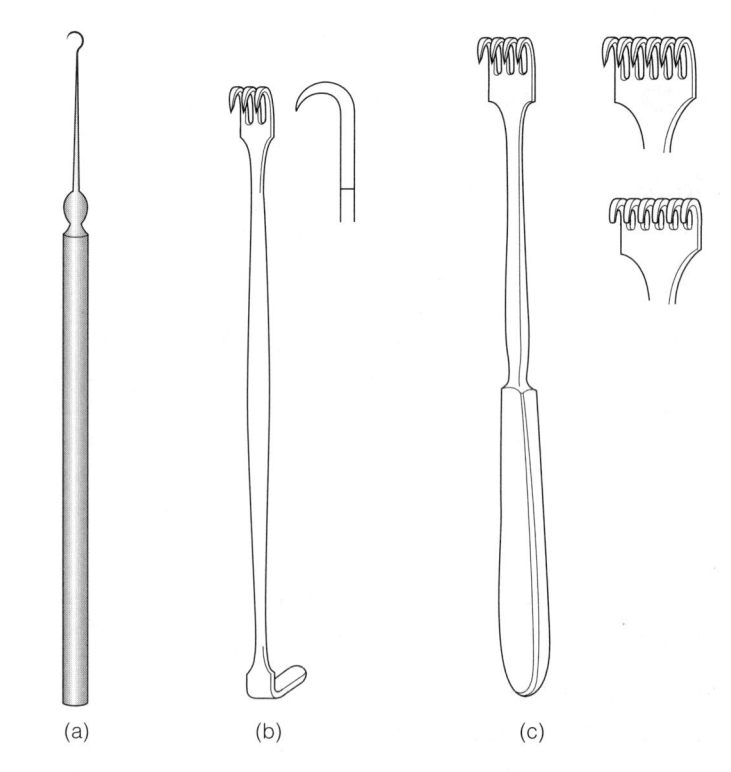

(a) Skin-hook retractor for the edges and corners of fine wounds
(b) Cats-paw retractor which also has a small flat blade
(c) A rake retractor which can have up to six sharp or blunt prongs

Fig. 2.39 *Small toothed retractors, hand-held*

Non-toothed small hand-held retractors

These include the Langenbeck retractor and the Durham-Barr retractor. They have a deeper blade which has specific usefulness in retracting subcutaneous tissue for minor skin surgery and body wall hernia surgery, and for subcutaneous fat retraction during deep wound closure (Fig. 2.40).

(a) Langenbeck retractor   (b) Durham-Barr retractor   (c) Czerny retractor

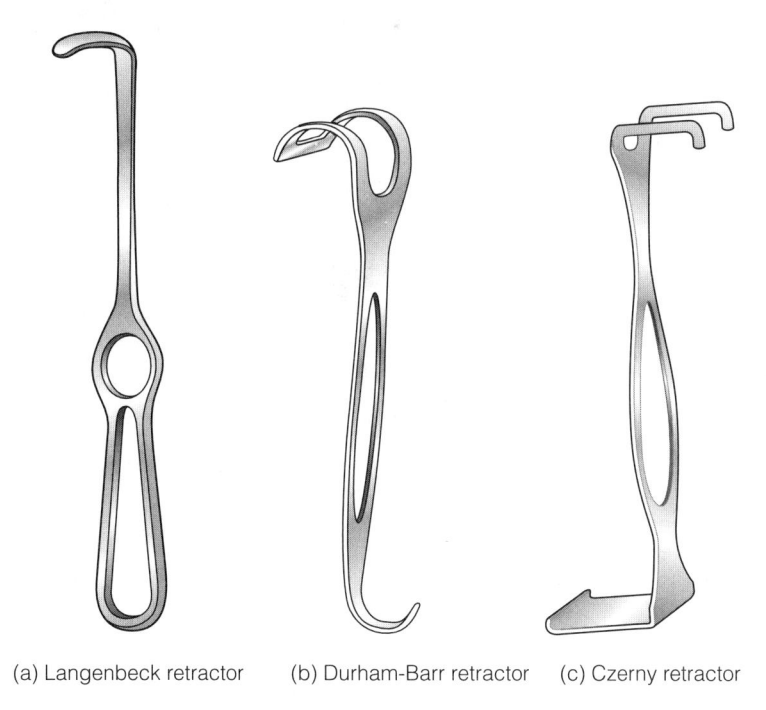

Fig. 2.40 *Small non-toothed (bladed) retractors, hand-held*

Large hand-held retractors
Superficial retractors

Superficial hand-held retractors are often quite wide with short blades. They may come with a curve (Fritsch or Kocher retractors) or a backward-pointing lip (Morris retractors) (Fig. 2.41). These patterns are used to great effect in retracting and lifting the anterior abdominal wall for better access into the superior, inferior and lateral recesses of the abdominal cavity. They are also used in axillary surgery and may sometimes be fixed to a self-retaining retractor for abdominal surgery (Fig. 2.46).

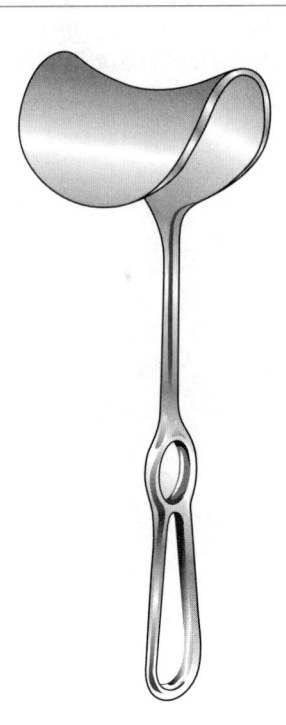

Fig. 2.41 *Fritsch retractor*

Deep retractors

Long, wide-bladed, hand-held retractors, of varying lengths, are excellent for retracting structures deep within the abdominal or thoracic cavities. The Deaver retractor is probably the best known (Fig. 2.42a) but other patterns include the St Mark's pelvic retractor (which may also have a light on it) (Fig. 2.42b) and the Kelly retractor. Great care must be exercised when using these retractors as their depth of penetration places adjacent structures, such as mesentery, liver or spleen, at risk of inadvertent damage. It is usually possible (and often advisable) to insert a gauze pack over the structure to be retracted as a protective buffer.

Self-retaining retractors

The common facet of self-retaining retractors is their ability to lock into a fixed position. Retention occurs by a system of springs, ratchets, screws, cranks or hooks. These retractors come in all sizes with toothed, flat or curved blades which may themselves be solid or fenestrated. Self-retaining retractors can be used in virtually any operative site but care needs to be taken as they provide a constant and potentially damaging pressure when applied. In some cases, a protective pack should be inserted between the retractor and tissues.

This category of retractor also incorporates the fixed position, multi-blade abdominal ring retractor systems.

(a) Deaver retractor   (b) St Mark's pelvic retractor

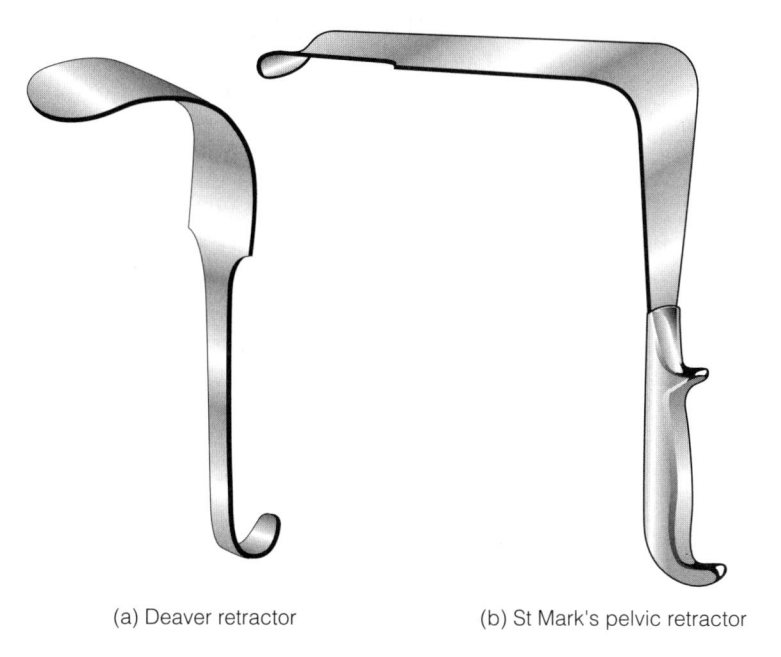

Fig. 2.42 *Heavy, deep, hand-held retractors*

Small self-retaining retractors

The smaller self-retaining retractors are generally used for cutaneous, superficial body wall or cavity (anal, vaginal and nasal) surgery. They come in several different patterns, most notably spring retractors, ratcheted retractors and screw-thread retractors.

Spring retractors

These are usually a thick wire-bodied retractor with teeth. The spring is a circle of wire at the base of the retractor which 'springs' the retractor out to a set distance. This type of retractor is only useful on fairly small wounds. The most common spring retractors have sharp teeth that are bent at right angles and embed within the tissues. This means that only structures such as fat and muscle should be retracted by them (Fig. 2.43).

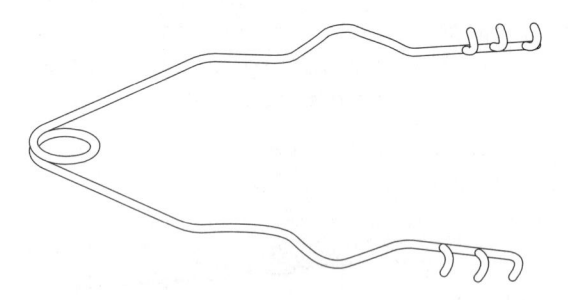

Fig. 2.43 *Spring retractor*

Ratcheted retractors

These retractors are usually scissor-pattern and may have a single hook, multiple teeth, flat blades or a combination of these with which to retract the tissues. One common pattern is the Weitlaner retractor (Fig. 2.44). They are of particular use in surgery on soft tissues, bones and fairly superficial structures including the anterior abdominal wall.

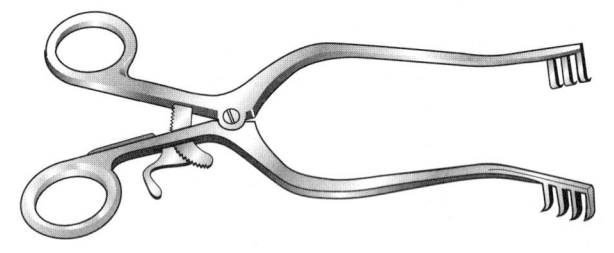

Fig. 2.44 *Weitlaner retractor*

Screw retractors

The most notable of this pattern is the Joll thyroid retractor (Fig. 2.45). Two clips, like towel clip heads (Fig. 2.53), are used to grip the dermis of the neck skin and the retractor is then wound out to retract the edges. The duck-billed vaginal speculum and some types of anal retractor also have screw mechanisms that open the blades and retain the position.

Large self-retaining retractors

The larger self-retaining retractors are used predominantly in deep-cavity surgery (abdomen and thorax), orthopaedics and various specific surgical procedures.

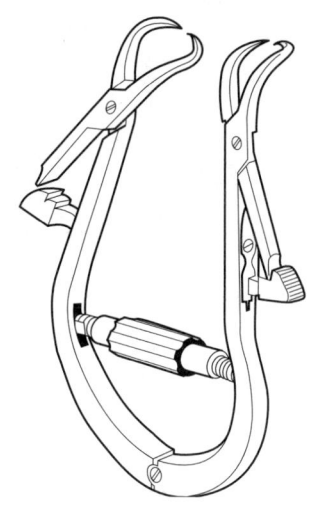

Fig. 2.45 *Joll thyroid retractor*

Screw retractors

In the context of a larger retractor the screw describes the mechanism of retaining the retractor's position while the actual opening and positioning is done by hand. Take, for example, the Balfour-Doyen self-retaining retractor (Fig. 2.46). Two long shafts with interchangeable fenestrated blades lie parallel, one of them sliding away from the other on a double rail system. The distance between the two arms is retained by a screw system or sometimes by friction alone. In between these blades a short body-wall retractor can be inserted to add pull at 90° to the major blades. This is also retained by a screw system (Fig. 2.46).

A variant of this system is the upper-hand retractor. A sterile transverse bar, with sliding attachments that carry a screw and wing nut, is secured to the table and lies within the sterile field. Various retractors can be screwed onto these attachments to provide fixed retraction, from above, in the upper abdomen (Fig. 2.47).

Crank retractors

Similar to the Balfour-Doyen, but without the extra blade, a Finichetto retractor has almost solid blades on the end of two heavy arms. A non-reverse rotating ratchet that must be actively cranked out to length and actively reversed to release the tension controls the distance between the two (Fig. 2.48). Because of its strength this retractor is used predominantly to spread ribs in thoracic surgery but may also be used in the abdomen.

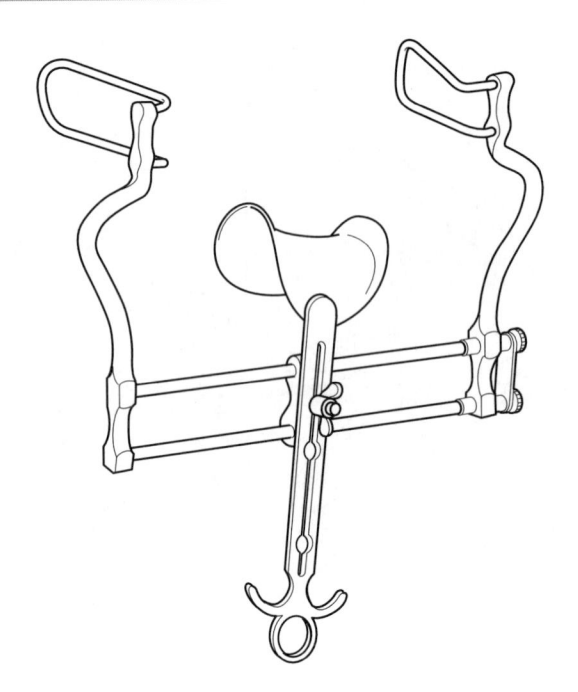

Fig. 2.46 *Balfour–Doyen retractor*

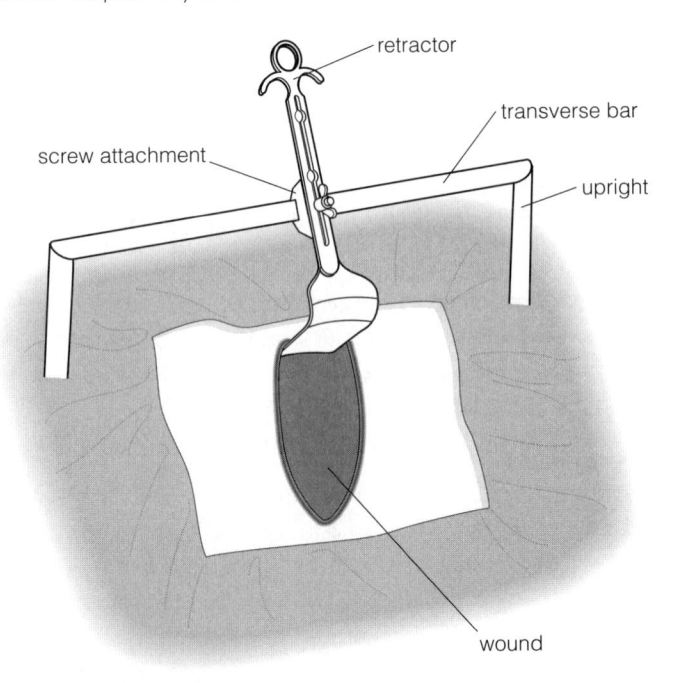

Fig. 2.47 *Upper-hand retractor*

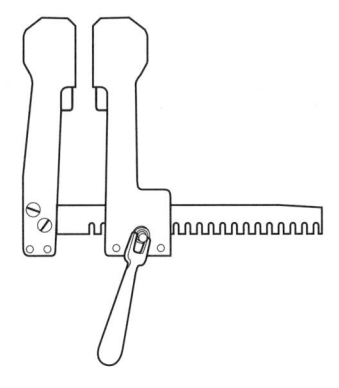

Fig. 2.48 *Finichetto retractor*

Hook retractors

These retractors are usually part of a complete abdominal retractor system in which a solid 'ring' is placed around the abdominal incision and retractors are hooked onto this ring to provide exposure. The retractor blades may be of any type.

There are two distinct types. In the first, the ring (which may be complete or incomplete) is secured to a sterile attachment which in turn is secured to the table but enters the sterile field. In this type, retractor attachments may be placed in any position. In the second type, the ring is free-standing and so the direction of pull exerted by each retractor attachment must counterbalance an opposing one in order to keep the system centralised (Fig. 2.49). Variants of this system are also used in neurosurgery.

Other instruments

There are several instruments that fit into no particular category but are important requirements of many operative procedures. These are items such as various designs of sucker, towel clips to hold the sterile drapes in place, and bowls in which to place fluids and objects.

Suckers

This group can be divided into the simple suckers in which all the material is sucked through a hole at the end of the single tube, and sump suckers in which air is mixed with the fluid to aid suction and prevent debris clogging the instrument.

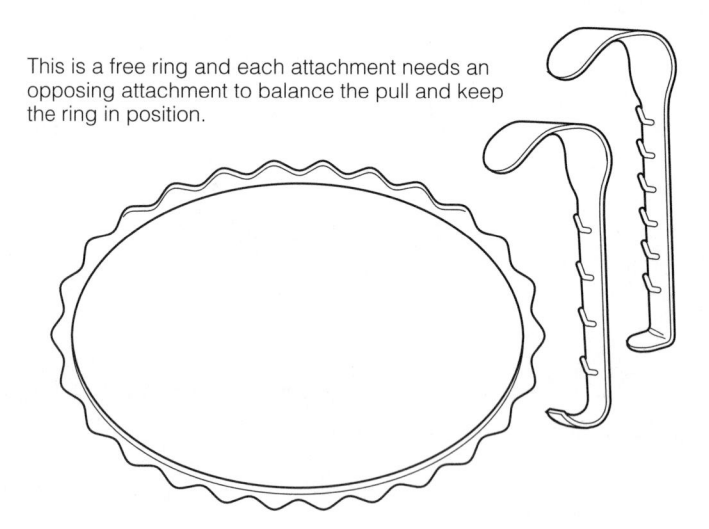

This is a free ring and each attachment needs an opposing attachment to balance the pull and keep the ring in position.

Fig. 2.49 *Denis Browne ring retractor*

Simple suckers

Small suckers

The typical ENT sucker is a perfect example of this. It has a small-calibre tube and a side hole that can be used to control the level of suction (Fig. 2.50).

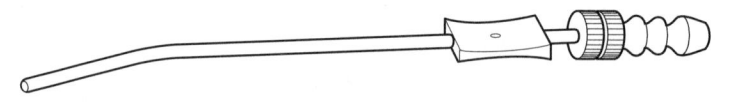

The American-pattern fine ENT-type sucker

Fig. 2.50 *ENT sucker*

Large suckers

The Yankauer sucker is longer and heavier than the ENT type, has an angled shaft and no side hole with which to control flow. The tip has a small screw-piece with four holes which limits what is sucked into the system. This is the most commonly used sucker in general surgery and comes in both metal and disposable plastic varieties (Fig. 2.51).

Sump suckers

This style of sucker has a simple central tube with a single end hole over which is screwed a sheath with multiple small perforations. This

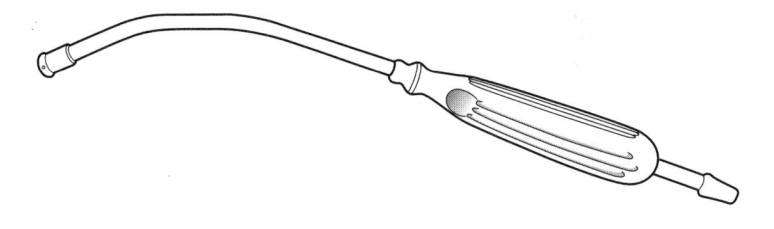

Fig. 2.51 *Yankauer sucker*

allows both fluid and air to be sucked into the gap between the two but prevents soft tissue or debris from occluding the system. Some variants have a button which turns the suction on and off as required. The Poole and Simpson-Smith suckers are two examples of this type (Fig. 2.52).

(a) Poole sucker

(b) Simpson-Smith sucker

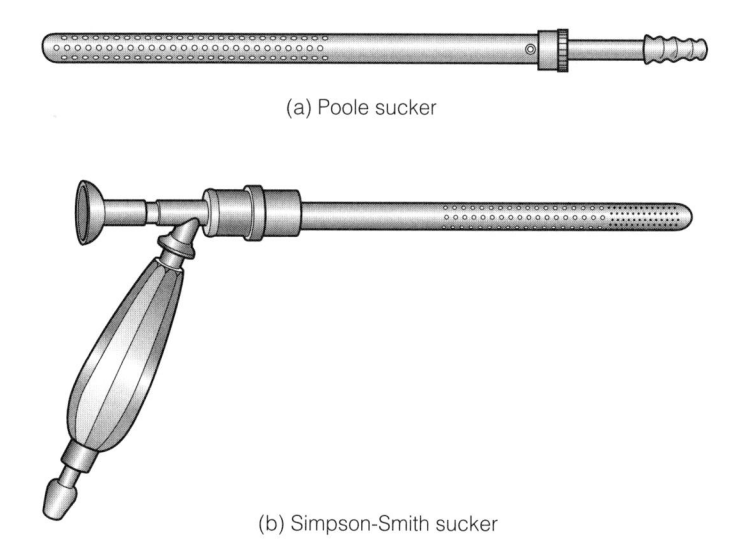

Fig. 2.52 *Sump suckers*

Towel clips

These are used to hold drapes, instrument scabbards, equipment leads and tubing in place. The two commonly used towel clips are a ratcheted scissor-pattern instrument, and a spring type that needs to be squeezed open and then returns passively to the closed position. Either type may have sharp, pointed or blunt and flat tips (Fig. 2.53).

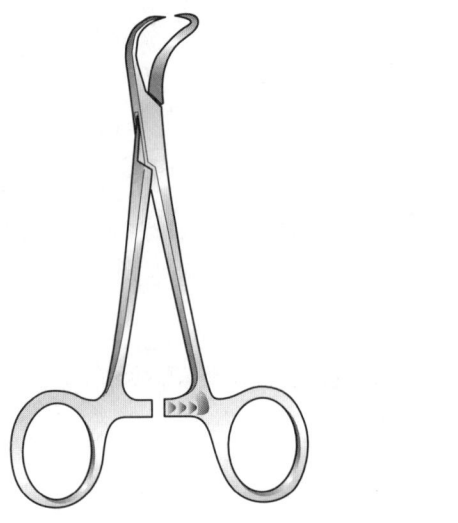

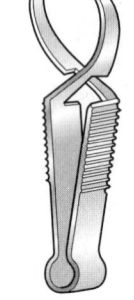

(a) Ratcheted scissors-pattern towel clip (b) Spring-action towel clip

Fig. 2.53 *Towel clips*

Bowls

Every sterile set needs bowls and kidney dishes of various sizes. Their uses include holding preparation solutions, passing sharps, holding wash or irrigation solutions, receiving specimens and collecting wound drainage, to name just a few (Fig. 2.54).

Surgical diathermy

Diathermy is an electrical device that can be used to coagulate bleeding from small-calibre blood vessels, and to cut through tissues. The basic principle of diathermy is that heat, created by the flow of current through tissues, will coagulate blood or vaporise tissue.

Diathermy has two modes—monopolar and bipolar. In the monopolar mode an electrosurgical generator is attached to the patient by a broad flat electrode and a live diathermy instrument is applied to the required site. The patient's body conducts the current between these two points to complete an electrical circuit (Fig. 2.55). In bipolar mode the active points are the two tips of a pair of insulated diathermy forceps and the current passes between them. The body does not make up part of the

(a) Kidney dish

(c) Jug

(b) Splash bowl for washing gloves in

(d) Gallipot (small) for preparation solution and other fluids

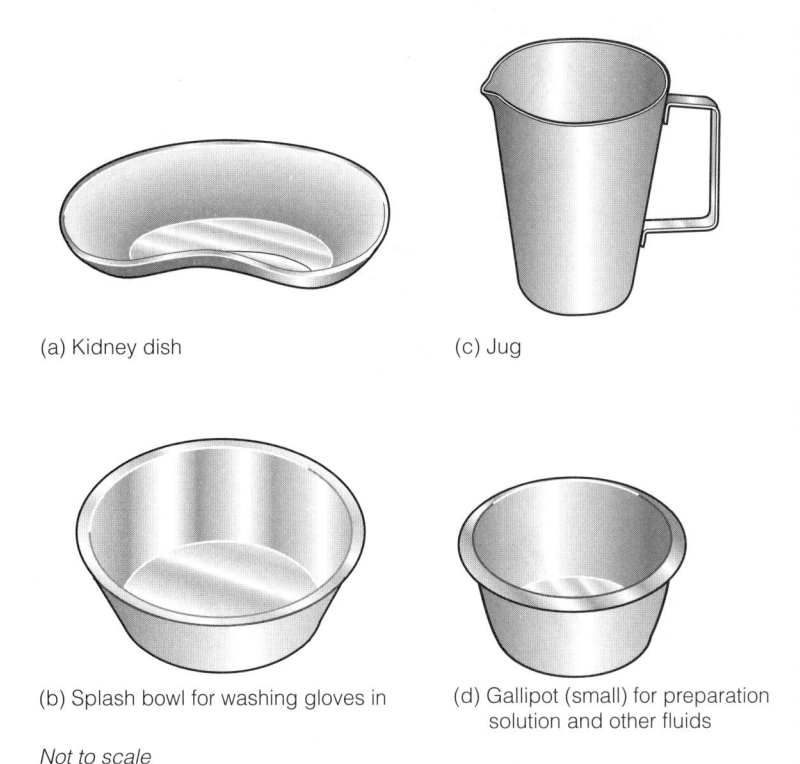

Not to scale

Fig. 2.54 *Containers*

circuit in bipolar mode and only tissue between the tips and immediately adjacent is heated (Fig. 2.56). Because of this local effect bipolar diathermy cannot be used to cut tissues.

The tissue effect produced by diathermy is directly related to the level of heat produced at the tip of the instrument. In monopolar diathermy the body makes up part of the electrical circuit and yet it is only at the instrument tip that the effect is needed. This introduces the concept of *current density*. For the greater part of its transit through the body, and at the electrode connected to the machine, the current is flowing through tissue with a broad cross-sectional area. Heat production here is minimal. As the area of current flow narrows (like a cone) at the tip of the diathermy instrument, the amount of current flow per unit of cross-sectional area of tissue (current density) increases. Consequently, heat production in this region increases rapidly to produce the desired effect (Fig. 2.57). Unfortunately, the current density can also become

Basic Surgical Skills

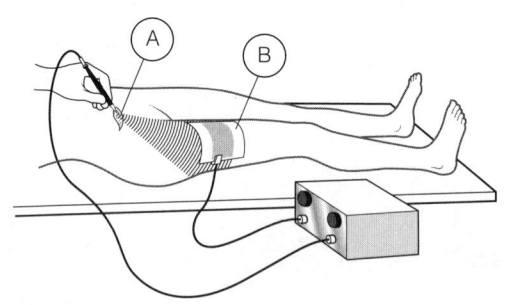

Current flows from the forcep at A to the plate at B and back through the machine. In this way the patient is an active part of the circuit.

Fig. 2.55 *Monopolar diathermy*

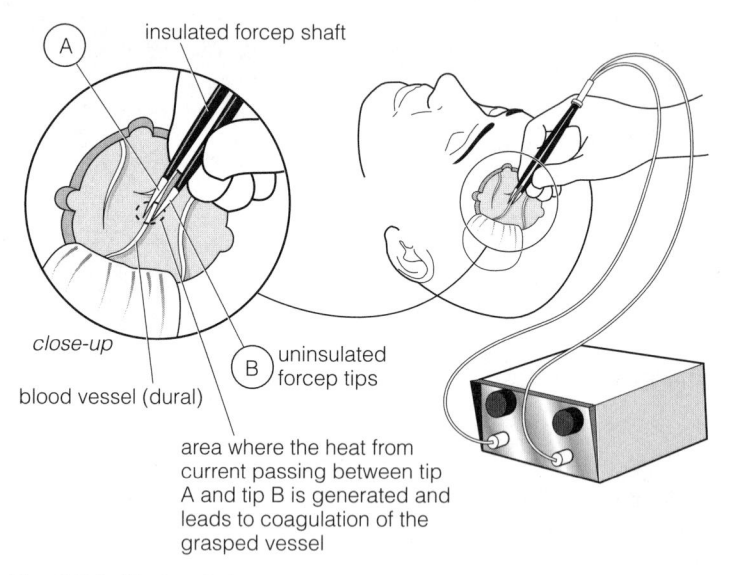

Fig. 2.56 *Bipolar diathermy*

very high if the current flows along fine pedicles, such as the cystic duct, or preferentially along small vessels or nerves in a digit. Inadvertent damage to these structures can happen and so diathermy should not be used if this situation may be a risk.

Monopolar diathermy

Monopolar mode allows current to run along lines of least electrical resistance to the plate electrode on the patient's skin. This must be large and have good electrical contact with the patient to reduce resistance

Basic Surgical Skills

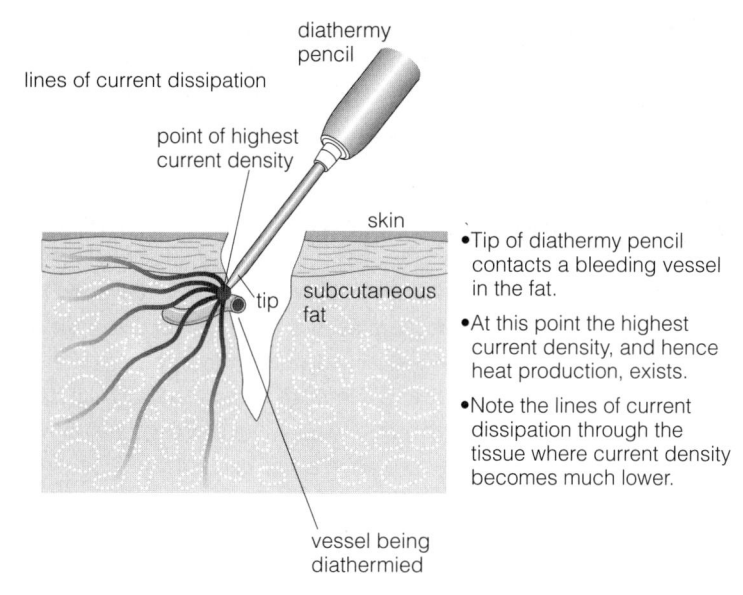

Fig. 2.57 *Current density*

Labels in figure:
- diathermy pencil
- lines of current dissipation
- point of highest current density
- skin
- tip
- subcutaneous fat
- vessel being diathermied
- Tip of diathermy pencil contacts a bleeding vessel in the fat.
- At this point the highest current density, and hence heat production, exists.
- Note the lines of current dissipation through the tissue where current density becomes much lower.

at this exit point. It is usually placed on the thigh, buttocks or back. Disposable gel electrodes are used and divided into two parts. A tiny current flows between these two parts to check adequate positioning of the electrode. If inadequate, an alarm will sound. Conversely, the point of contact between the diathermy tip and the patient should be small and dry. This maximises current density and therefore increases the efficiency and level of heat production.

The electric current that is generated is of very high frequency (0.5 to 2 Mhz) and so, unlike household electricity at 50 hz, is too fast to affect the electrical system of the heart. For each type of diathermy the 'strength' of the current can be adjusted in order to produce higher levels of energy. It may even be so high as to arc between the patient and the electrode, thereby producing wide surface charring called *fulguration*. This is an excellent method of haemostasing oozing surfaces.

A variant on the standard electrode is the argon beam diathermy. In this instrument the current is carried down a spray of argon gas. This spreads over a wide surface and both fulgurates the surface and coagulates down the line of superficial vessels.

Within the monopolar mode two types of current can be generated. The cutting current is a continuous waveform that produces very high temperatures and vaporises tissue. The coagulation waveform is produced as intermittent bursts of energy and, while this will vaporise tissue, it also flows along vessels to coagulate the blood within them and stop bleeding. Both of these can be used on virtually any tissue except bone.

Bipolar diathermy

Bipolar mode relies on the passage of alternating current between the two tips of an insulated instrument as they close on a piece of tissue. This is an excellent way to seal small vessels with minimal surrounding tissue damage, as no current flows through these tissues. This makes bipolar diathermy the method of choice for neurosurgery, ophthalmology and when operating on digits and the penis.

Further reading

Friedin J & Marshall V. *Illustrated Guide to Surgical Practice*, Churchill Livingstone, Melbourne, 1984. Chap. 4, The Operation.

McGregor A & McGregor I. *Fundamental Techniques of Plastic Surgery*, 9th edn, Churchill Livingstone, Edinburgh, 1995. Chap. 3, Free Skin Grafts.

Thompson RVS. *Primary Repair of Soft Tissue Injuries*, Melbourne University Press, Melbourne, 1969. Chap. 3, Basic Instruments for Outpatient Reparative Surgery.

Suture materials and surgical needles

CHAPTER THREE

Surgery of virtually every type has a common element in the use of threads for suturing (sewing) and ligating (tying and securing). Many materials have been used over the centuries for these purposes including such bizarre items as giant ant heads (the bodies being ripped off after the bite had closed the wound), vegetable fibres wound figure-of-eight around giant thorns passed through both wound edges, and sterilised barbwire in Japanese POW camps.

Modern sutures comprise a range of highly refined materials that have undergone rigorous testing. Some are specifically designed for the purpose of suturing alone. Most are attached (*swaged*) to a needle and are presented in sterile packaging for use in one patient only. Constant demand on the suture industry for improved performance, and a combination of better and cheaper materials, has led to huge advances in suture and needle technology. This chapter introduces suture materials and the needles on which they are loaded.

Of equal importance to understanding suture materials is a knowledge of suture sizes and needles. A great variety of needles are available, already attached to the suture (*swaged needles*) or available for threading with loose individual threads (*eyed needles*). The size, shape and curve, tip and cross-sectional profile are what determine the major functions of a needle and these are dealt with in the next section.

Surgical needles

Needles are an integral part of suture technology and an understanding of their basic concepts will facilitate appropriate use. Most are made from corrosion-resistant stainless steel and attached to their thread by a *swage*—a pre-drilled hole at the base of the needle into which the thread is bonded. Needles must be rigid enough to penetrate the tissue without bending, ductile enough to deform without breakage and as slim as possible without being weak. The point must be sharp enough to penetrate tissues reliably and big enough to carry the suture with minimal tissue trauma. The needle must also be of a three-dimensional shape that permits secure handling within the needle holder, without the risk of slippage and subsequent tissue trauma.

Table 3.1 Desirable properties of a surgical needle

1. Corrosion-resistant material, e.g. stainless steel
2. Rigid enough to penetrate tissue without bending
3. Ductile enough to deform without breaking
4. Slim enough to cause minimal trauma to tissues
5. Wide enough to draw the thread through tissue without undue abrasion
6. Sharp enough to penetrate tissues easily
7. A method of thread attachment, e.g. eye or swage
8. Stable when grasped and used in an instrument

Source: Compilation assisted by information from *Wound Closure Manual*, published independently by Ethicon Inc. 1994

Anatomy of a surgical needle

A standard set of terms is used to describe the common features of a surgical needle. *Needle point* and *swage* are self-explanatory. *Chord length* is the straight-line distance from the point to the swage. *Needle length* is the distance from point to swage when measured around the needle's outer surface. *Radius* is the distance from the centre of a circle, of which the needle describes an arc, to the needle itself. *Needle diameter* is the thickness of a needle at any part of the *needle body* (see Fig. 3.1).

Surgical needle characteristics

The most important characteristics of surgical needles are:

- shape and curvature
- needle length and wire diameter (size)

Basic Surgical Skills

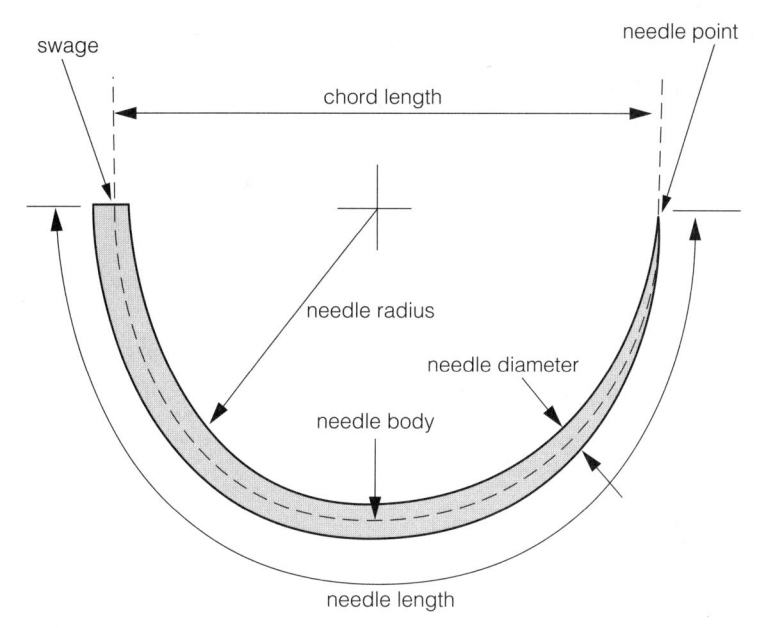

Fig. 3.1 *Characteristics of a surgical needle*

- tip and cross-sectional shape
- attachment to the suture material

Shape and curvature

The shape and curve of a needle will often dictate its function. Certain specialised needles are used for specific circumstances, e.g. J-shaped, (Fig. 3.2).

1/4 circle—Ophthalmic and microsurgery
3/8 circle—General use in all tissues
1/2 circle—General use in all tissues
5/8 circle—CVS and cavities (oral, nasal, pelvis, umbi, etc.)
Straight—General use (but discouraged as hand-held)
J-shaped—Similar to 5/8 (femoral hernia)

Needle length and wire diameter (size)

The potential length of a needle is dictated by the thickness of wire used, and the principle features of rigidity, ductility and strength will guide the needle size that can be formed. Obviously, a 66 mm needle of ultra-thin wire gauge will bend or break far too easily to be of any use and the same applies (but less so) for very short thick-diameter needles. Long needles tend to be used for fascia and skin closure with

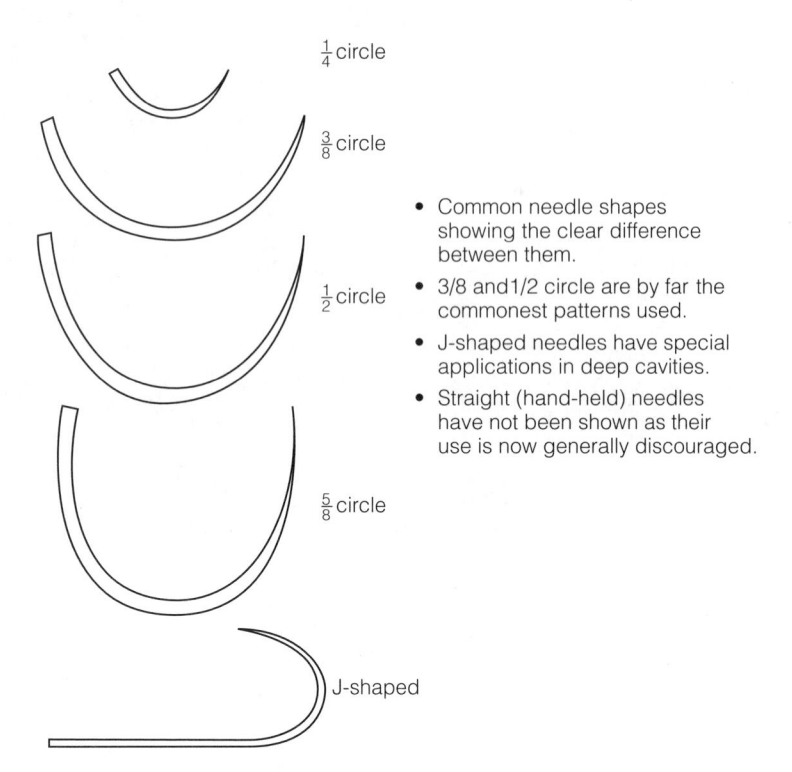

Fig. 3.2 Needle shapes and curves

- ¼ circle
- ⅜ circle
- ½ circle
- ⅝ circle
- J-shaped

- Common needle shapes showing the clear difference between them.
- 3/8 and 1/2 circle are by far the commonest patterns used.
- J-shaped needles have special applications in deep cavities.
- Straight (hand-held) needles have not been shown as their use is now generally discouraged.

heavier gauges of wire and hence heavier sutures. Shorter and finer needles have uses in visceral, vessel or fine structure surgery. In the same way, thickness of wire should match the functional requirements of the stitch, the suture it carries and the length of the needle.

Tip and cross-section

The point of a needle is that part from the extreme tip to the maximum cross-sectional diameter. From here back the body may retain the same shape or it may change. There are four main point types: cutting (conventional), reverse cutting, taper point and blunt.

The main tip type encountered is one with a sharp, pointed profile. **Conventional cutting** and **reverse cutting** needles are sharp and pointed with a triangular cross-section. They cut through tissue and so are used mainly on skin, periosteum, tendons and sclera. The *upwards facing cutting edge* on the conventional cutting needle gives it a tendency to incise upwards into tissue while using a standard suturing technique. This may result in sutures tearing through the tissue being repaired. The reverse cutting needle, which has the cutting edge on the outer curve, presents a *flat edge forwards* and so is unlikely to cut out. The latter is the more commonly used of these two (Fig. 3.3).

There are several variations of the cutting point, such as the spatula, diamond and lancet points. These all have specialised functions and are not dealt with here.

Taper-point needles have a round body that tapers to a sharp point. They penetrate initially with this sharp tip but then push (or split) the tissues apart with the round body. This works well with viscera and most fascia but tough, often high-collagen containing tissues such as skin, tendon and scar are not as amenable to this type of needle. Taper-point needles will penetrate these tissues but the excessive force required and the resultant tearing of tissues make it a vastly inferior pattern in these situations. Variations also exist on the tapering needle with a combination of a cutting point and a tapering round body forming the taper-cut needle.

Blunt needles are the second major needle profile and have been developed as a variation of the taper point for safety reasons. They have a standard tapering, circular body cross-section with a point that is gently rounded at the tip. As this is quite fine it will still penetrate fascia easily but is far less likely to penetrate glove material or skin. The round needle body then passes as a normal taper-point needle by splitting tissues. Their use is particularly in liver repair and vascular regions where they will slide past (not penetrate) vessels, and in safer fascial closure with respect to the potential for needlestick injuries.

Needle bodies may retain the same cross-section for their entire length or may flatten out on the inner and outer curves to facilitate grasping by a needle holder. Some needles have roughening or grooves on them to improve the grip further and some are siliconised for even smoother penetration.

Attachment to suture materials

Needles usually come preattached to their threads. The technology to allow this has been developed only in the last few decades. Traditionally, all needles were eyed and the threads were inserted by the scrub-nurse prior to use. Eyed needles are still manufactured but are rarely used except in gynaecology and unusual circumstances. See Figure 3.4.

Reverse cutting (edge down)

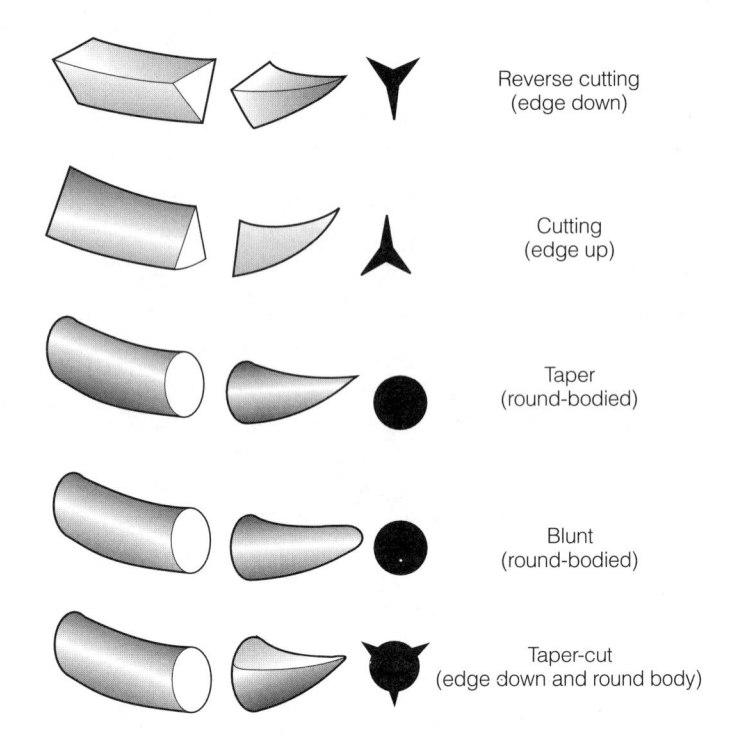

Cutting (edge up)

Taper (round-bodied)

Blunt (round-bodied)

Taper-cut (edge down and round body)

Fig. 3.3 *Shapes of needle points and bodies showing body cross-section, tip shape, and the defect created in the sutured tissue by the needle*

Preattachment, or swaging, may be accomplished in two ways. In the first a hole is drilled in the end of the needle, the suture is inserted into this and the end is pressed in (crimped) on four sides to secure it. In the second method, a split is made down the centre of the needle and the suture is inserted. The two sides are then crimped together to hold the suture in place.

There are several advantages to swaging. It allows minimisation of tissue trauma as the thread is virtually the same size as the needle rather than having a double thickness of thread as in an eyed needle. There is a potential reduction of leakage at anastomotic sites as the thread fills the entire needle hole. This is especially useful in vascular surgery. Convenience is improved, as needles no longer have to be threaded. This serves the additional purpose of minimising needle handling.

Basic Surgical Skills

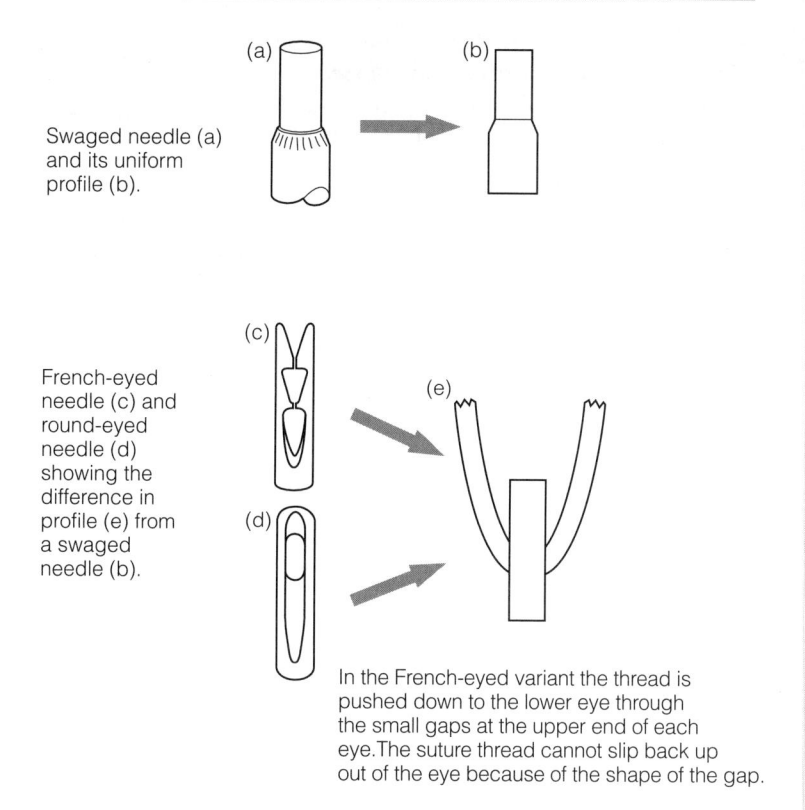

Swaged needle (a) and its uniform profile (b).

French-eyed needle (c) and round-eyed needle (d) showing the difference in profile (e) from a swaged needle (b).

In the French-eyed variant the thread is pushed down to the lower eye through the small gaps at the upper end of each eye. The suture thread cannot slip back up out of the eye because of the shape of the gap.

Fig. 3.4 *Swages and eyes*

Suture sizes

The sizing of sutures initially followed a pattern set by the United States Pharmacopeia (USP standard). This classification related to the minimum and maximum diameters of the material in inches and the minimum knot pull strength. Different standards were required for organic absorbable sutures and other (non-absorbable and synthetic absorbable) sutures (see Tables 3.2 and 3.3).

In competition with the USP system there exists a European Pharmacopeia (EP) system based on millimetre thickness and different knot pull tests. This is also known as the metric system (see Table 3.4).

The most commonly used suture sizes would be in the range of 5/0 to 1 (when looking at general surgery). Tissues that are thicker, or more collagen-rich, require larger sutures and heavier needles (see Table 3.5). Sizes outside this standard range would usually be reserved for specialty

Table 3.2 USP standards for catgut
(USP standard, organic absorbable materials)

Size	Diameter Min. (in.)	Min. (mm)	Max. (in.)	Max. (mm)	Minimum limit for knot pull strength (lbs)	(kp)
9/0	.0007	0.018	.0015	0.038	0.05	0.023
8/0	.0015	0.038	.0025	0.064	0.10	0.045
7/0	.0025	0.064	.0035	0.089	0.13	0.06
6/0	.0035	0.089	.0050	0.127	0.35	0.16
5/0	.0050	0.127	.0070	0.179	0.70	0.32
4/0	.0070	0.179	.0095	0.241	1.5	0.68
3/0	.0095	0.241	.0125	0.318	2.5	1.13
2/0	.0125	0.318	.0160	0.406	4.0	1.81
0	.0160	0.406	.0195	0.495	5.5	2.50
1	.0195	0.495	.0230	0.584	7.5	3.40
2	.0230	0.584	.0265	0.673	9.0	4.08
3	.0265	0.673	.0300	0.762	11.5	5.22
4	.0300	0.762	.0340	0.864	13.0	5.90
5	.0340	0.864	.0385	0.978	16.0	7.26

Source: *Wound Closure—Materials and Techniques*, published independently by Davis and Geck 1990

practice such as plastics, ophthalmology and orthopaedics. Sutures under 6/0 in size (human-hair diameter) require some magnification (loupes or microscope) to be used effectively. They are utilised mostly for microvascular work or plastic microsurgery. An excellent account of suture sizes is found in the Davis and Geck™ wound closure manual written by Zederfeldt and Hunt (Fig. 3.5).

Suture materials

The main properties of each suture material can be classified within three broad categories: first, the origin of the material, second, the type of strand produced and, third, the pattern of breakdown in tissues.

Suture materials may either be a *natural substance* (silk, linen or catgut) or a *synthetic polymer* (polypropylene, polyester or polyamide). The production of any suture material results in either a single, solid

Table 3.3 USP standards for materials other than catgut (USP standard, nonabsorbable materials and synthetic absorbable materials)

	Diameter				Minimum limit for knot pull strength			
	Min.		Max.		Class I*		Class III**	
Size	(in.)	(mm)	(in.)	(mm)	(lbs)	(kp)	(lbs)	(kp)
10/0	.0005	0.013	.0010	0.025	0.09	0.04	0.11	0.05
9/0	.0010	0.025	.0015	0.038	0.11	0.05	0.13	0.06
8/0	.0015	0.038	.0020	0.051	0.20	0.09	0.24	0.11
7/0	.0020	0.051	.0030	0.076	0.31	0.14	0.35	0.16
6/0	.0030	0.076	.0040	0.102	0.51	0.23	0.60	0.27
5/0	.0040	0.102	.0060	0.152	0.99	0.45	1.20	0.54
4/0	.0060	0.152	.0080	0.203	1.50	0.68	1.80	0.82
3/0	.0080	0.203	.0100	0.254	2.50	1.13	3.00	1.36
2/0	.0100	0.254	.0130	0.330	3.50	1.59	4.00	1.80
0	.0130	0.330	.0160	0.406	5.00	2.27	7.50	3.40
1	.0160	0.406	.0190	0.483	7.00	3.17	10.50	4.76
2	.0190	0.483	.0220	0.559	7.40	3.85	13.00	5.90
3	.0220	0.559	.0250	0.635	10.00	4.54	16.00	7.26
4	.0250	0.635	.0280	0.711	12.50	5.67	20.00	9.11
5	.0280	0.711	.0320	0.813	16.00	7.26	25.00	11.4
6	.0320	0.813	.0360	0.914	20.00	9.1	30.00	13.6
7	.0360	0.914	.0400	1.016	25.00	11.3	35.00	15.9

*Class I = silk, synthetic absorbable and nonabsorbable sutures
**Class III = stainless steel

Source: Wound Closure—Materials and Techniques, published independently by Davis and Geck 1990

monofilament (nylon, polydioxanone or polypropylene) or a multifilament strand that has been either twisted (catgut) or braided (polyester or silk). The breakdown characteristics of a suture material are broadly absorbable (catgut, polydioxanone or polyglycolic acid) or nonabsorbable (nylon, polyester and stainless steel) although there is some overlap with substances such as silk which will eventually undergo degradation in tissues.

While origin and absorption are self-explanatory, the need to distinguish between monofilament and multifilament should be explained. Monofilament sutures excite far less tissue reaction than multifilament

Table 3.4 EP (metric) standards compared with USP standards

USP size codes Organic absorbable materials	USP size codes Nonabsorbable materials and synthetic absorbable materials	EP size codes (mm) Organic and synthetic absorbable material. Nonabsorbable materials	Suture diameter (mm) Min. Max.
	11/0	0.1	0.01–0.019
	10/0	0.2	0.02–0.029
	9/0	0.3	0.03–0.039
	8/0	0.4	0.04–0.049
8/0	7/0	0.5	0.05–0.069
7/0	6/0	0.7	0.07–0.099
6/0	5/0	1	0.10–0.14
5/0	4/0	1.5	0.15–0.19
4/0	3/0	2	0.20–0.24
3/0	2/0	2.5	0.25–0.29
2/0	0	3	0.30–0.39
0	1	4	0.40–0.49
1	2	5	0.50–0.59
2	3	6	0.60–0.69
3	4	7	0.70–0.79
4	5	8	0.80–0.89
5	6	9	0.90–0.99
6	7	10	1.00–1.09

Source: *Wound Closure—Materials and Techniques*, published independently by Davis and Geck 1999

sutures and do not harbour the microorganisms that collect in the irregularities on a multifilament suture's surface. Multifilaments may be either a simple twisted thread (such as catgut) or a true braided thread (such as silk). This means that infection and scarring are much reduced with the use of monofilament sutures (Fig. 3.6).

These three characteristics are probably the most important constant properties of materials used for suturing. Other attributes such as initial

Table 3.5 Suture selection

Size	Comparison	Uses
12/0 (to 7/0)	Four times smaller than a human hair	Exclusively microsurgical
6/0	Human-hair size; generally the smallest suture used with naked vision	Face, blood vessels
5/0		Face, neck, blood vessels
4/0		Mucosa, neck, hands, limbs, tendons, blood vessels
3/0		Limbs, trunk, gut, blood vessels
2/0		Trunk, fascia, stomach, viscera, blood vessels
0–1	Small pencil lead	Abdominal wall closure and other heavy fascial uses

tensile strength, stretch, handling qualities, knotting characteristics, the body's reaction to the material and strength degradation rate are all either variable with environment and conditions or of no benefit in classification (see Table 3.6, at end of chapter).

In general absorbable sutures leave no residue and are used on tissues where healing will take place quickly and continued tissue strength will not depend on the strength of the suture material e.g. subcutaneous tissue, ties on vessels etc. Nonabsorbable material is required for tissues which are slow to heal or require continued suture strength for their stability. Where reduced tissue reaction or avoiding infection is desirable, such as in skin or deep fascial closures, a monofilament should be used. The compromise of slow absorbing monofilaments, such as polydioxanone, give advantages from both groups.

Many of the suture materials, such as linen, cotton, stainless steel or silk are either rarely used or only have a role in certain specific areas. While these are excellent materials they often have cheaper or better alternatives available from the synthetic classification set.

Percentage volumetric reduction with decreased size of suture

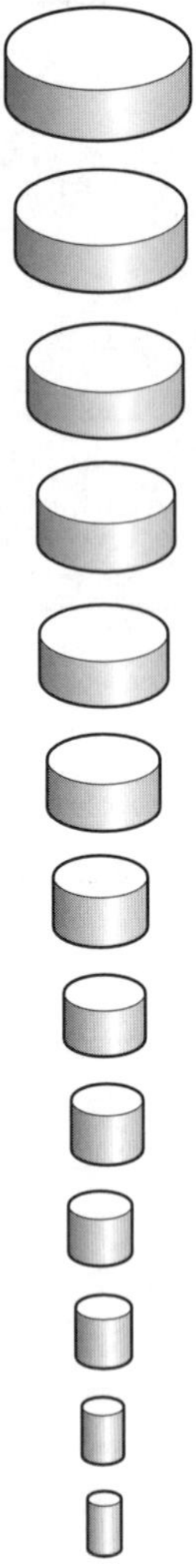

USP	EP	mm	% reduction
3	6	0.60–0.69	
2	5	0.50–0.59	28
1	4	0.40–0.49	33
0	3.5	0.30–0.39	31
2/0	3	0.25–0.29	27
3/0	2	0.20–0.24	51
4/0	1.5	0.15–0.19	40
5/0	1	0.10–0.14	49
6/0	0.7	0.07–0.099	54
7/0	0.5	0.05–0.069	50
8/0	0.4	0.04–0.049	44
9/0	0.3	0.03–0.039	40
10/0	0.2	0.02–0.029	50

Fig. 3.5 *Relative suture sizes and reductions*

Properties of common suture materials

Catgut

Natural, multifilament and absorbable

Catgut is produced from sheep gut submucosa or beef gut serosa. It is split, twisted, dried and polished to a monofilament profile and may

Basic Surgical Skills

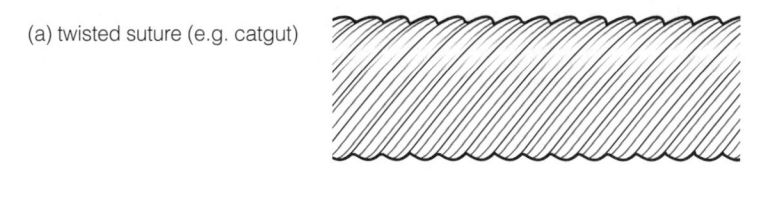

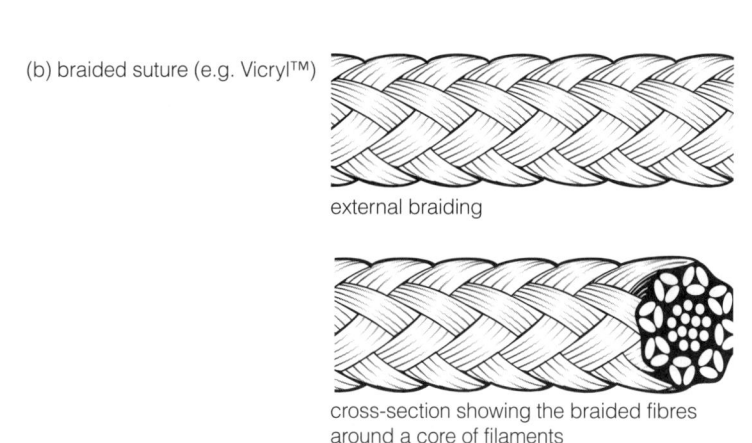

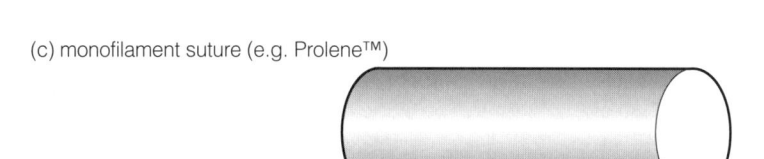

(a) twisted suture (e.g. catgut)

(b) braided suture (e.g. Vicryl™)

external braiding

cross-section showing the braided fibres around a core of filaments

(c) monofilament suture (e.g. Prolene™)

Fig. 3.6 *Suture materials*

also be chrome tanned to delay absorption. Catgut is digested by proteolytic enzymes from phagocytic cells in 80–120 days and promotes a marked tissue reaction. There is little tensile strength left by 10 days and this loss may be even quicker (24 hours) when used in the stomach or ileum. Chromic gut takes about twice this time to lose strength.

Catgut comes in sizes 7/0 to 3 (USP) on cutting, round-bodied or taper-cut needles, and as free ties or on a dispensing reel. It must be stored in fluid medium or the suture dries out and becomes rigid (except Davis and Geck **Softgut**™ which is dry-packaged). Gut sutures have considerable 'memory' and require straightening before use. They dry out rapidly once opened and are prone to fraying. Once dry, catgut can be quite difficult to tie.

Catgut should only be used when long-term wound strength and support is not required. Use is contraindicated in cardiovascular and neurological tissues.

Common use
- subcuticular and subcutaneous sutures
- liver sutures
- appendiceal stump/oversew
- urinary tract
- mesentery

Polyglycolic acid (PGA)
Synthetic, multifilament and absorbable

A polymer of glycolic acid, its monofilament form is too brittle for use, so the extruded filaments are stretched and braided to attain high tensile strength. **Dexon II**™ is stronger, loses less strength in knotting and excites less inflammatory reaction than catgut. PGA hydrolyses from the 10th to 90th day in a predictable and uniform way. Suture strength is lost over 3–4 weeks.

Tissue drag and abrasion due to braiding is alleviated by coating the suture with a dry lubricant but this reduces knot security. As there is little slip in this material when it is knotted, the first throw of each knot must be placed with precise tension and accuracy. It is produced in sizes 5/0 to 2 and is available on a wide range of needles. It is used in many similar situations as catgut but retains strength longer and so has several other applications.

Common uses
- GI anastomosis
- muscle and fascial closures
- subcuticular skin closure (undyed suture)

Polyglactin 910
Synthetic, multifilament and absorbable

A cousin to polyglycolic acid, **Vicryl**™ is a copolymer of glycolide and lactide. The braided filaments are coated with a mix of polymer and calcium stearate to reduce drag. Absorption, by hydrolysis, commences at around 20–40 days and is complete by 60–90 days. There is some inflammatory reaction, as with PGA, and the strength and knotting are also very similar. Strength is lost over a 3–4 week period. Vicryl comes in a wide range of sizes (8/0 to 2) and needles.

Common uses
- GI anastomoses
- muscle and fascial closure
- subcuticular skin closure

Trimethylene/Glycolic acid
Synthetic, monofilament, absorbable

The monofilament polymer, **Maxon**™, is synthetic and therefore non-antigenic and non-pyrogenic. There is minimal tissue reaction and patient discomfort. Non-enzymatic hydrolysis is uniform in all patients and is generally completed between the 180th and 210th days. Maxon has a high tensile strength (28 lb straight pull), loses half of this over 5–6 weeks in a predictable pattern, and thus has long-term wound support characteristics. Being monofilamentous it has good tissue running and knot slip characteristics. It is available from 7/0 to 2 in a full range of needles.

Common uses
- GI anastomoses
- fascial closure
- caesarean section

Polydioxanone
Synthetic, monofilament and absorbable

The polyester polymer, **PDS II**™, is heat extruded into monofilaments. Although absorbable, strength at implantation is very high. There is little pyrogenicity or antigenicity and tissue reaction is minimal. Absorption by hydrolysis starts at 90 days and is complete by 6 months. PDS II exhibits good handling but usually requires four throws to hold well. It is useful in slow-healing areas but infection markedly accelerates loss of strength. It can also be made into clips and staples which are absorbed and therefore do not affect magnetic resonance imaging. The suture is available in 6/0 to 2 on a full needle range.

Common uses
- GI anastomoses
- fascial (abdominal) closure
- subcuticular (skin) closure

Poliglecaprone 25

Synthetic, monofilament and absorbable

The newest absorbable synthetic, **Monocryl**™, is a copolymer of glycolide and caprolactone. It has good tissue run characteristics, being a monofilament, and handles and ties well. The polymer is non-antigenic and pyrogenic with little tissue reaction. Its absorption profile is predictable (fully absorbed between 91 and 119 days) and all tensile strength is lost by 21 days. It is available in sizes 5/0 to 1 in a range of needles.

Common uses
- subcuticular (skin) suture
- ligation
- subcutaneous suture

Polybutester

Synthetic, monofilament and nonabsorbable

A polymer, **Novafil**™ is very supple with good handling and tying characteristics. It excites minimal reaction in tissues. There is low tissue drag, good knot rundown and first throw security. Tensile strength is high and it has permanent tissue retention. Its unique property is marked elasticity and recoil to original size without permanent distortion or damage. It is available in 10/0 to 2 and on a full range of needles.

Common uses
- skin closure (plastics)
- ophthalmology
- fascial closure (general)

Polyvinylidene

Synthetic, monofilament and nonabsorbable

Similar in nature to polypropylene, **Vilene**™ is a minimally reactive monofilament suture. No other information is available at present.

Common uses
See *polypropylene* below.

Polyether

Synthetic, monofilament and nonabsorbable

Described as similar to polybutester, **Dyloc**™ is a minimally reactive stretchable monofilament suture. No other information is available at present.

Common uses
See *polybutester* above.

Polyamides
Synthetic, multi/monofilament and nonabsorbable

Nylon is usually a monofilament but may be braided. It has poor handling and knotting qualities and thus requires multiple throws and knot burying. There is a lot of 'memory' and some loss of strength over time but minimal absorption or breakdown. It is also available in many sizes (10/0 to 2) and virtually all needle types.

Common uses
- fascial (abdominal) closure
- skin closure
- hernia surgery
- vascular surgery
- neurosurgery

Polypropylene
Synthetic, monofilament and nonabsorbable

Another non-reactive polymer, with minimal tissue reaction, **Surgilene**™ (Davis and Geck) and **Prolene**™ (Ethicon) have high tensile strength like nylon with less weakening and far less memory. These properties make general use and knotting far easier. It also has good knot security and loses virtually no strength over time. Available in 10/0 to 2 on all needle types, Surgilene/Prolene is a popular suture choice.

Common uses
- fascial (abdominal) closure
- vascular anastomoses
- subcuticular (skin) closure
- tendon repairs
- ophthalmology

Polyester
Synthetic, multi/monofilament and nonabsorbable

Yet another polymer, polyester has high and permanent tensile strength and excites minimal tissue reaction. Most companies have a variety. It has excellent handling and tying characteristics with good knot security

Table 3.6 Suture materials: a classification

Breakdown	Origin	Strand	Generic name	Trade name
Absorbable	Natural	Multifilament	Catgut—plain	}GENERIC
			Catgut—chromic	}KNOWLEDGE
				}ONLY
		Monofilament	None	}Most companies
				}have a variant
	Synthetic	Multifilament	Glycolic acid polymers	
			—polyglycolic acid	**Dexon**™ (D+G)
			—polyglactin 910	**Vicryl**™ (Ethicon)
				Polysorb™ (USSC)
		Monofilament	Polydioxanone	**PDS**™ (Ethicon)
			Trimethylene / Glycolic acid	**Maxon**™ (D+G)
			Poliglecaprone 25	**Monocryl**™ (Ethicon)
Nonabsorbable	Synthetic	Multifilament	Polyester	**Ethibond**™/**Mersilene**™ (Ethicon)
				Ti-Cron™/**Dacron**™ (D+G)
				Dyflex™/**Teflex**™/**Polyflex**™ (Dynek)
			Polyamide (nylon)	**Surgilon**™ (D+G)
				Nurolon™ (Ethicon)™

Suture materials and surgical needles

Monofilament	Polyamide (nylon)	**Ethilon**™ (Ethicon) **Dermalon**™ (D+G) **Nylene**™ (Dynek)	
	Polypropylene	**Prolene**™ (Ethicon) **Surgilene**™ (D+G)	
	Polyvinylidene	**Vilene**™ (Dynek)	
	Polybutester	**Novafil**™ (D+G)	
	Polyether	**Dyloc**™ (Dynek)	
Natural Multifilament	Silk	} GENERIC	
	Linen	} KNOWLEDGE	
	Cotton	} ONLY	
	Stainless steel	} Most companies	
Monofilament	Stainless steel	} have a variant	

(D+G) Davis and Geck, a division of Cyanamid, US
(Ethicon) A division of Johnson & Johnson Medical
(USSC) United States Surgical Corporation, parent company of Autosuture
(Dynek) An Adelaide-based Australian-owned suture company

after 5–6 throws. In monofilament form there is some gauged elastic recoil. To improve tissue run the multifilament is coated with silicon or teflon. The fibre is also woven into vascular grafts. Comes in sizes 6/0 to 1 in all needle types.

Common uses
- cardiac valve surgery
- tendon suture
- orthopaedics
- ophthalmology

Silk/Cotton/Linen
Natural, multifilament and nonabsorbable

Used less commonly in the 1990s due to the available alternatives. Silk is still frequently used by older surgeons who have never found a better handling alternative. It is easy to handle but loses strength by enzymatic digestion because, like cotton and linen, it is a protein. All three excite marked inflammatory reactions. They come in a range of sizes from 5/0 to 1 on all needle types.

Common uses
- skin closure
- vascular ligation
- GI anastomosis
- ophthalmology
- cardiac surgery

Stainless steel
Natural, multi/monofilament and nonabsorbable

Once again a rarely used suture, stainless steel retains great strength and excites minimal response. Tissue passage is good but 'knot tying' is difficult—in fact, it is most commonly twisted together and bent over. This is the strongest of all suture materials and comes in sizes 4/0 to 7 on a limited range of needles.

Common uses
- sternal closure
- hernia (shouldice repair)
- contaminated wounds
- orthopaedics

Further reading

Friedin J and Marshall V. *Illustrated Guide to Surgical Practice*, Churchill Livingstone, Melbourne, 1984, 1st edn. Chap. 4, The Operation, pp. 133–7.

Zederfeldt H and Hunt T. *Wound Closure—Materials and Techniques*, Davis and Geck, USA, 1990.

Thomson S. *Super Suturing*, Davis and Geck, Australia, 1991.

Ethicon. *Wound Closure Manual*, Johnson & Johnson, USA.

The last three books are available through the hospital representatives of Ethicon and Davis and Geck.

Basic surgical skills

Basic principles and the operative field

Since the earliest records of surgery hundreds of methods of repairing tissues have been described. Any technique will only be successful if the surgeon follows a set of basic prerequisites applicable to all levels of surgical competence.

Understanding and attitude

The surgeon must be acutely aware of the aims of the procedure, of how it is performed, the limitations it has and its pre-, peri- and post-operative care. Surgeons should aim to work in a calm situation and attempt to remain composed at all times. Goals and objectives must be set and modified in relation to the desired outcome, the simplest effective solution and the ability of the patient to tolerate this. The unexpected should be evaluated in light of the aims of the procedure and, if necessary, changes made to the operative plan.

Exposure and positioning

The incision and the operative field, as defined by the visible area within the drapes, must both be large enough to allow easy and comfortable access for all steps of the operation. Surfaces within the draped sterile field should also be kept tidy and clean to prevent suture tangling, component damage and undue delay. Adequate anaesthesia should keep the patient relaxed and so improve access to deep structures that require mobilisation and repair.

Surgeons should plan every manoeuvre and adjust their position to perform each one with maximum ease. This may require only rotation of the shoulders, but grosser adjustments such as sitting or moving to the other side of the patient may be needed. It is wise to practise both unfamiliar manoeuvres and familiar ones in unusual positions, thereby learning appropriate motor patterns. In times of doubt or stress the basic principles should be strictly adhered to.

All people have a resting tremor and this is exacerbated by the anxiety of operating. To minimise the effect of this tremor both instruments and hands can be steadied against a firm base. This may be as simple as resting an elbow on the table to steady the forearm complex or bracing the operating hand against the patient or the other hand. Instruments such as scissors can be balanced against fingers of the opposite hand to ensure stability while cutting.

Lighting the operative field

Bright, concentrated light should illuminate all parts of the operative field but be directed primarily onto the area where tissue is being manipulated. The assistant should alter the lighting to best effect and this will usually be required multiple times during a procedure. Do not be afraid to use a headlight or lighted retractor for working in deep cavities.

Maintenance of the operative field

The site of operation and its surrounds are generally referred to as the 'operative field'. There are certain conventions to be followed regarding the construction and maintenance of this field but by ensuring *sterility* and *tidiness* the likelihood of a procedure's success will be improved. These two principles are dealt with next, from the practical viewpoint of *preparing and draping* the patient and *instrument placement*.

Preparing and draping the operative site

This refers to the preparation of the operative field by the application of antimicrobial solutions to the site of operation (prepping) and the exclusion of other areas with sterile towels or sheets (draping).

Common preparative solutions include chlorhexidine (0.5%) in alcohol (70%), chlorhexidine (0.5%) and cetrimide (2%), 10% povidone-iodine solution, alcoholic iodine solution and aqueous chlorhexidine (0.5%) (see Table 6.3). All these have a bactericidal action and all but the aqueous chlorhexidine have some amount of 'detergent' activity to overcome the natural oils on the skin. This helps the solution 'stick' to the patient. Special care must be exercised when using diathermy after alcoholic preparations. The surgeon must ensure that all the alcohol has evaporated or a spark may cause it to ignite. This is a well-documented complication that occurs virtually every year somewhere in Australia.

When scrubbed, a member of the operative team will 'paint' the operative site with a skin preparation solution. This should start at the site of incision and go outwards in a spiral fashion. Swabs used for prepping should be discarded when dry and a new one used, not the old one re-dipped. A wider area than required should be prepped to allow for potential wound extension in unforeseen circumstances.

The 'drapes' used to create a sterile field may be made of cotton, paper or plastic. They are held in place by a combination of gravity, friction and towel clips. In some situations a large adhesive plastic sheet is applied to the entire field to secure the drapes and cover the skin prior to incision. Some of the disposable drapes have an adhesive layer that sticks them to the patient. If waterproof drapes are not used a plastic sheet is placed between the drapes and the patient. This is to protect the patient and to prevent complete 'soak-through' which is theoretically a break in sterile technique.

Drapes are applied and secured after 'prepping' is completed. In general the whole patient (except the head) is covered with drapes, and two-layer coverage is the minimum standard at any point on the patient. A raised sterile curtain is usually placed between two IV poles to separate the anaesthetist and the surgeon (known colloquially as the 'blood–brain barrier'). This protects both from contamination but is not practical in head or neck surgery. Draping techniques will not be dealt with in this manual as they are intensely specific to each specialty and are often further personalised by each surgeon.

Instrument issues

Most of the instruments required for an operation will be stored on trolleys controlled by the scrub-nurse. Instrument safety is improved by use of the concept that all instruments and sharps are 'owned' by the scrub-nurse. This means that the surgeon is merely 'borrowing' them and that they must be returned personally to their owner, not just dropped in the operative field or on the patient. This will ensure that all instruments are accounted for and that no sharps are left in an unexpected position, thus increasing the safety of the patient and operative team.

The only instruments that belong on the operative field are the diathermy, sucker, instrument scabbard and any clamps or self-retaining retractors while *in situ*. Unfortunately, the last two may catch other instruments, hands or threads, resulting in damage to tissues or tangling. To minimise this annoyance and risk, exposed instruments can be steadied and protected by covering them with an opened wet pack.

The theatre environment

Operative surgery is a stressful and dangerous undertaking and the absolute responsibility for any procedure's success belongs to the surgeon alone. The comfort and priorities of the surgeon, then, should dictate the conduct of other theatre personnel during a procedure. Distractions such as conversation and music should be kept to a minimum unless specifically requested and the surgeon's concentration (especially at a vital juncture) should not be broken by unnecessary interruptions. This applies equally to the anaesthetist who may require silence for concentration on a particularly difficult situation before, during or after the operation. Always err on the side of quietness if in doubt.

Tissue blood supply

No matter what tissue is being repaired the absence of oxygenated blood from the site of healing will cause healing failure. The presence of free arterial bleeding within a wound, or at the end of a segment of bowel, is the absolute indicator of viability. Conversely, blanching and cyanosis with dark venous ooze indicates an inadequate initial blood supply and likely failure of repair that is performed.

One of the adverse consequences of surgical repair is that initially viable tissue may be compromised and then fail to heal. Traumatic tissue-handling techniques, suture line tension, devascularisation during mobilisation, strangulation with overtight knots and excessive haemostatic diathermy to the cut surfaces may all play a part in this process.

Conversely, excessive bleeding can lead to wound haematoma formation. This is a factor in the development of wound infection and disruption. A balance must be achieved, then, between the two extremes to provide a non-bleeding but viable wound.

Tension in the wound

Tension is the arch-enemy of surgical healing as it leads to mechanical disruption due to distracting forces, ischaemia due to increased tissue pressures and the potential for necrosis and infection at the wound edge. Care must be taken to appose tissues loosely, except where a watertight seal is required. Mobilisation of tissues and preservation of their vascular supply is vital in preventing both ischaemia and mechanical disruption of the wound. This principle applies equally to all tissues and in all branches of surgery.

Assistance during the procedure

Skilled assistance is invaluable. Anatomy will be best displayed, tensions maintained and other conditions optimised by operating with an assistant who understands the procedure being performed. Without this, mistakes can be made and the result may be suboptimal for the patient. Experience derived while assisting an experienced practitioner is also an ideal way to learn and appreciate operative surgery.

Summary

This section has dealt with some of the practical and philosophical issues that need to be understood by all practitioners undertaking procedures. They will be differentially important depending on the type of procedure and situation but all have some level of application in every procedural situation. Reflection on these points will not directly improve manual skills but may well improve the conduct, and even success, of an individual procedure.

Basic suturing techniques

This section deals with basic suturing techniques used in the repair of skin and fascial planes. Without this skill it is virtually impossible to carry out any form of surgery. The combination of dexterity, instrument handling, tissue handling and the exposure to tissue tension make suturing and knot tying the perfect introduction to surgical skills. While other structures may also require sutured repairs it is beyond the scope of this basic skills manual to deal with these.

Introduction to suturing tissues

Some basic conventions apply to the suturing of all tissues. *Round-bodied*, or *taper*, needles are used for fat and fascia and *reverse cutting* or *cutting* needles for skin. The needle should be grasped in a needle-holding forcep (see Chap. 2) of appropriate size. Tissues such as the skin edge should be handled lightly with a fine to medium toothed forcep, of Adson or Gillies pattern, or a skin-hook, to avoid crush damage. This same principle, with appropriate tools, applies to all types of tissues for suturing. The width and distance between sutures depends on the suture material, the tissue and the site of the wound. In general terms the suture should run as deeply as the distance from the skin edge to the suture entry point. The sutures should be spaced as widely as the distance from entry hole to exit hole, thereby forming squares (Fig. 4.1a).

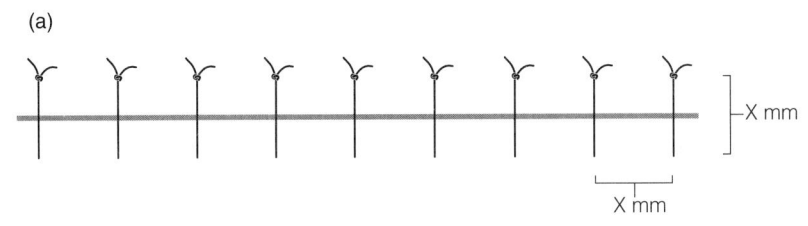

(a)

Sutures along a wound are spaced at approximately equal intervals (X mm). This corresponds with the width of the stitch and allows the sutures to form a square (box) pattern.

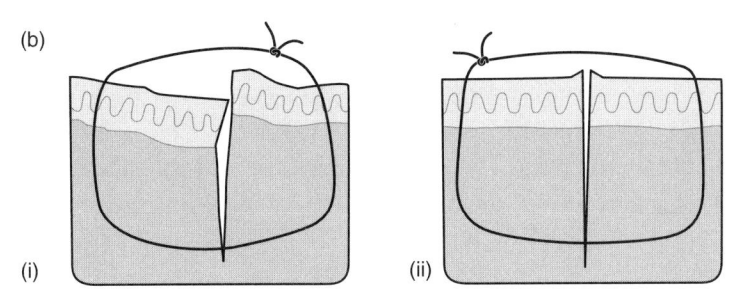

(b)

Demonstration of placing the knot on the side of the wound that allows the skin to sit most evenly. When on the right (i) the skin is uneven but if the knot is moved to the left (ii) this evens out.

Fig. 4.1 *Placement of sutures*

When inserting sutures one must take care to balance them evenly. Equal bites must be taken on each side of the wound and the knot laid to the side of best sit (Fig. 4.1b). Interrupted (individual) sutures should be equally spaced and the tag ends cut so as not to touch the next suture (Fig. 4.1a). The stitch itself should not grossly indent the skin at insertion, just loosely but accurately appose tissue, as postoperative swelling will cause each one to cut into epidermis and leave scarred 'train-tracks'. If excessive pressure is caused, ischaemia may supervene, leading to wound-edge necrosis and potentially serious infections. These factors apply equally to deep tissues. Excessive dead space allows for haematoma formation and infection, but tight sutures will themselves strangulate and necrose fat, muscle and fascia, also providing a nidus for infection and wound weakness.

The most commonly used suture materials for interrupted and exposed skin sutures are nylon and **Prolene**™. These are non-absorbable, synthetic monofilament fibres and usually need to be removed between the 5th and 10th postoperative days, depending on the site. Sutures that are buried, or run in the skin as the subcuticular does, may use either nonabsorbable sutures as above or absorbable materials such as catgut, **Vicryl**™, **Dexon**™ or **Monocryl**™ as an alternative. There are exceptions to these basic rules, which apply in certain clinical settings, but these basic options will safely cover all common situations.

Simple suture

As the name suggests, the simple suture (Fig. 4.2) is the basic pattern of suture and the one on which all others are based. It is useful in many situations and must be the major tool in any surgeon's suturing armoury.

The curved needle should be gripped in the tips of the forceps, two-thirds of the way from the point to the swage, and enter the tissue (skin) at 90°. It should traverse a *virtually* semicircular course to exit skin again at 90°. This is often performed in two separate bites, each describing a 90° arc. Once the needle enters the bottom of the wound it should be removed, reinserted into the holder and the second arc begun from the depths of the wound.

The knot is tied and adjusted to give the best 'vertical' apposition of skin edges. If more deep tissue than superficial is taken the skin edges will evert. Similarly, if less is taken the edges will invert. This pattern of suture may also be used in deep tissues with the knot either buried or superficial (Fig. 4.2).

Basic Surgical Skills

(a)

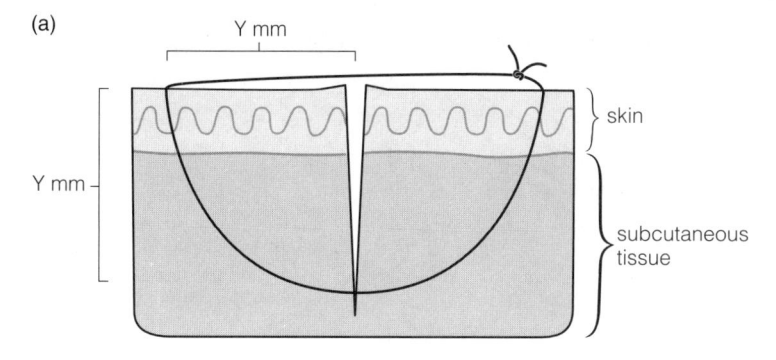

A schematic representation of the semi-circular simple suture. The depth of the bite and the distance from skin puncture site to the centre of the wound are both a 'radius' in distance (Y mm) and should be virtually equal.

(b) Three variants of the simple suture

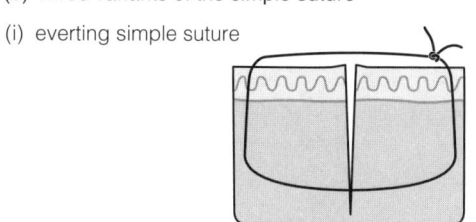

(i) everting simple suture

The everting simple suture picks up more subcutaneous tissue than the skin width and, when tied, this deeper tissue is squeezed superficially to evert the edges of the wound.

(ii) inverting simple suture

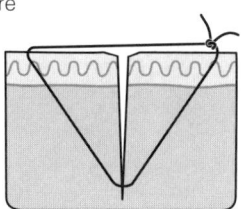

The inverting simple suture does the opposite of (i) and takes less deep tissue. This allows the more superficial tissues to roll in towards each other causing inversion. A suture like this should not be used in skin but is very useful for inverting bowel edges in anastomoses.

(iii) buried simple suture

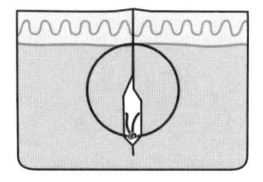

The buried simple suture is used to secure deep layers of tissue and approximates a circle rather than a semi-circle.

Fig. 4.2 *Simple suture*

(c) Inserting a simple suture

(i) The skin edge is lifted back and the needle is inserted at 90° to the skin

(ii) With a pronating action of the forearm the needle is driven through the tissues in a semi-circular course to exit in the depths of the wound

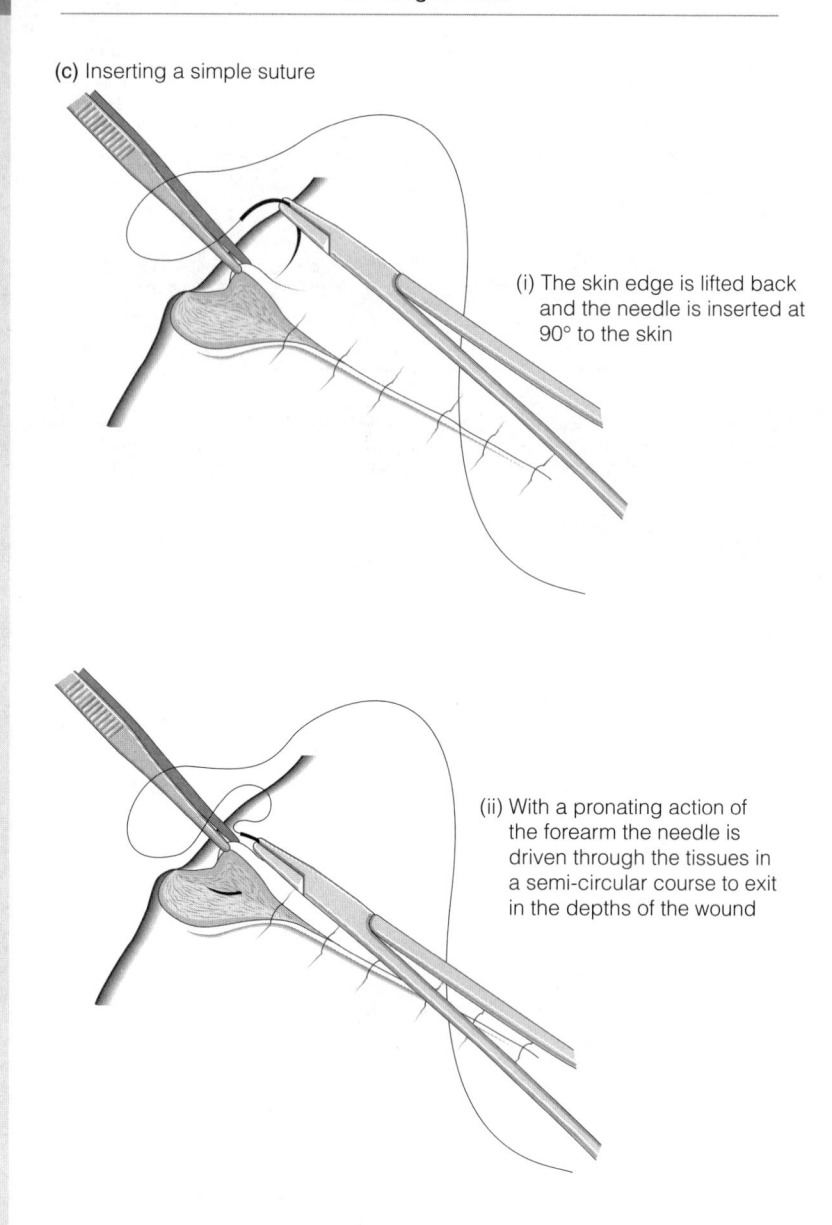

Fig. 4.2 *Simple suture (cont.)*

Basic Surgical Skills

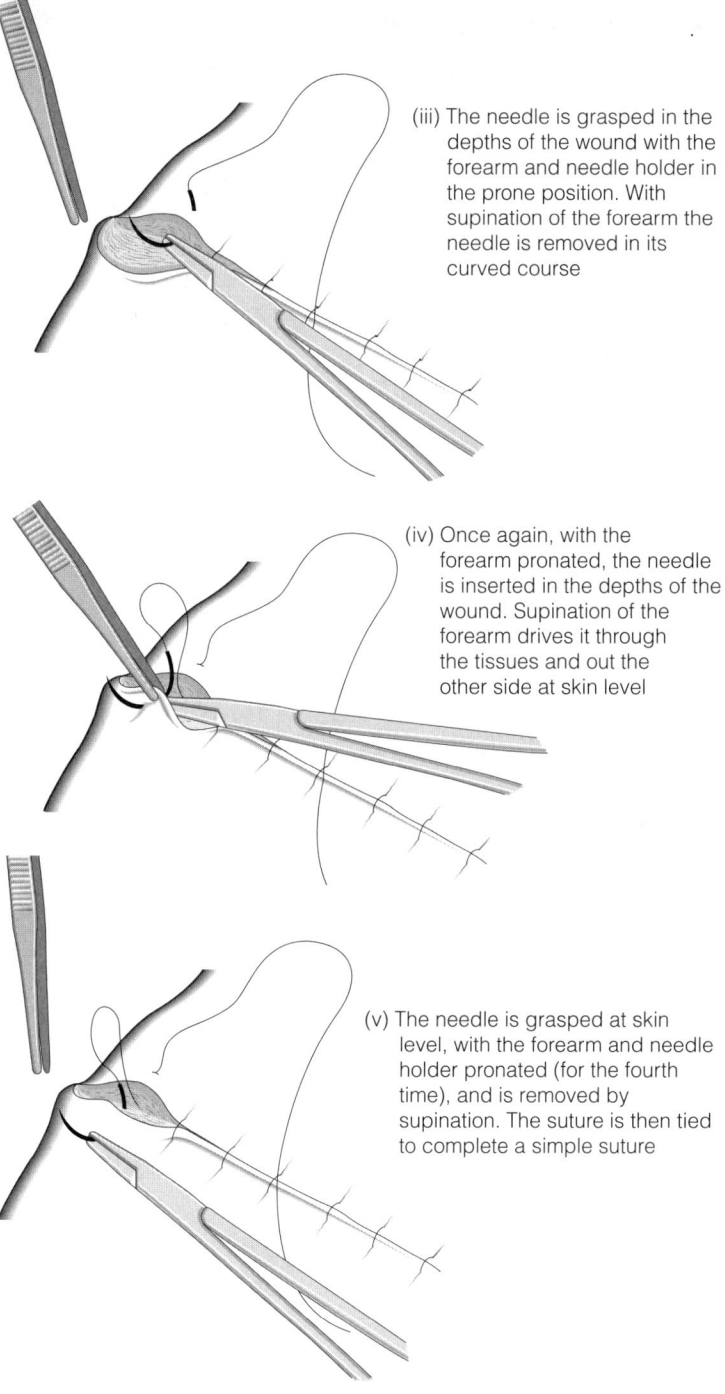

(iii) The needle is grasped in the depths of the wound with the forearm and needle holder in the prone position. With supination of the forearm the needle is removed in its curved course

(iv) Once again, with the forearm pronated, the needle is inserted in the depths of the wound. Supination of the forearm drives it through the tissues and out the other side at skin level

(v) The needle is grasped at skin level, with the forearm and needle holder pronated (for the fourth time), and is removed by supination. The suture is then tied to complete a simple suture

Fig. 4.2 *Simple suture (cont.)*

Vertical mattress suture

The vertical mattress suture (Fig. 4.3) is almost the same as a simple suture but, after the needle has exited the skin, it is reversed in the needle holder and reinserted to pick up just the skin (epidermis and dermis) of both wound edges. This second small set of bites is in the same line as the original stitch (Fig. 4.3a). This ensures eversion of the edges and better healing. This suture is best used in creases and areas of natural inversion (e.g. the back of a hand or other sites of loose skin). To reduce ischaemia it may be alternated, on a 1:1 or 1:2 basis, with simple sutures.

The major potential problem with this suture is that it can cause excessive pressure on the tissues. If the sutures are so close and tight that they prevent dermal blood flow this may subsequently cause skin-edge ischaemia and necrosis. Luckily, this complication is rare.

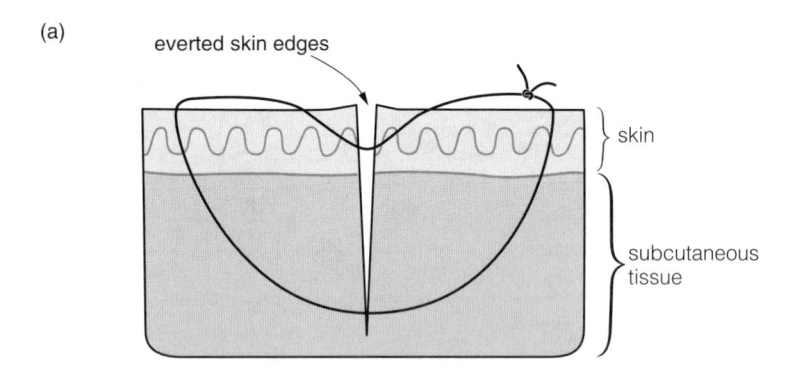

(a)

A schematic representation of the vertical mattress suture showing how the skin is picked up with a second 'mini-suture' in the same line as the main suture. This ensures eversion of the skin edges.

Fig. 4.3 *Vertical mattress suture*

Basic Surgical Skills

(b) Inserting a vertical mattress suture

The first five steps correspond with Figures 4.2(c)(i) to (v).

(vi) The needle is reversed in the needle holder and the edge of the skin, in the same line as the main suture, is picked up

(vii) Moving the forearm from mid prone to fully prone drives the needle through the tissues

(viii) The skin on the opposite side of the wound is picked up to complete the mattress suture and the suture is tied

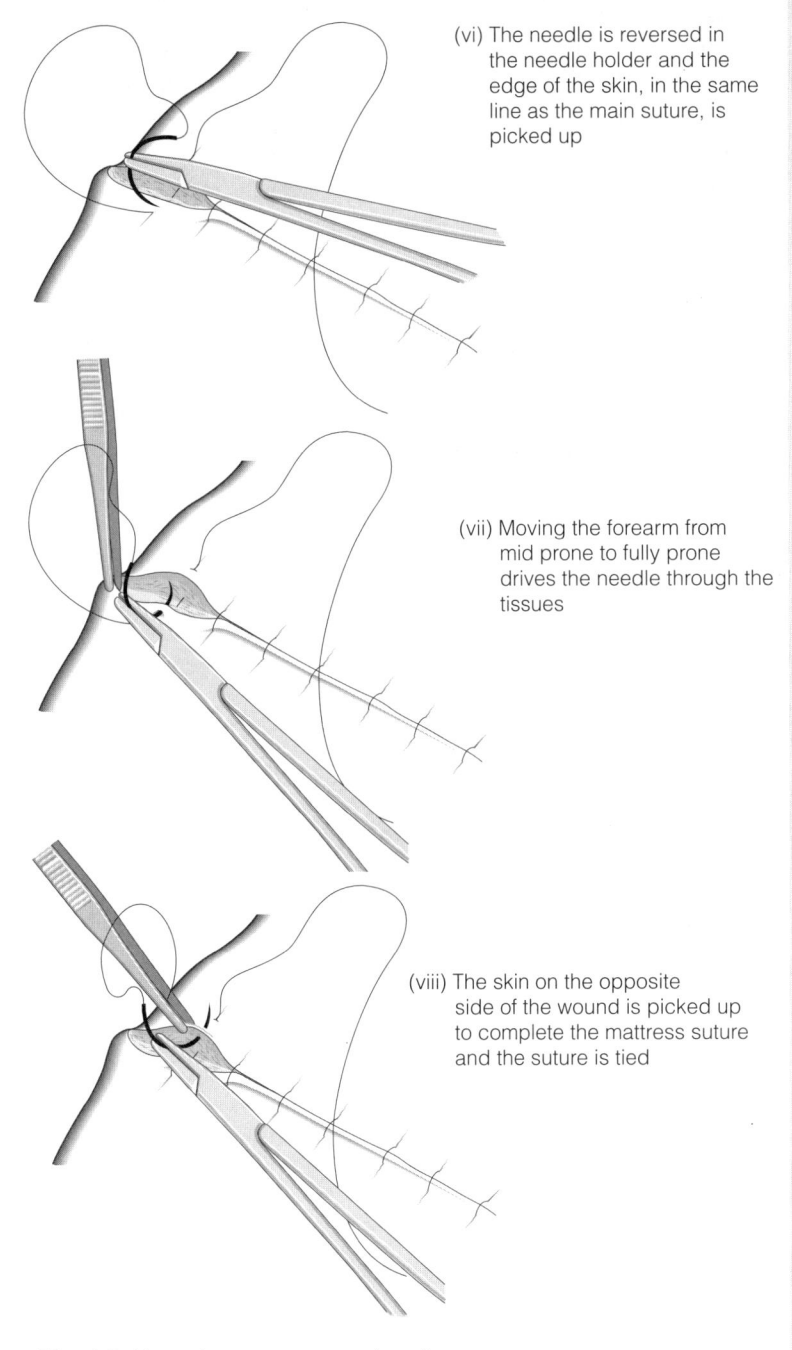

Fig. 4.3 *Vertical mattress suture (cont.)*

Horizontal mattress suture

The horizontal mattress suture (Fig. 4.4) is also useful for ensuring eversion of the skin. In essence it is two parallel simple sutures which, instead of being tied individually, are inserted with the one thread. They have a bridge of suture joining them on one side of the wound and the two tied ends on the other. When inserting the horizontal mattress suture it starts as a simple suture and then the needle is reversed as in the vertical mattress variant. At this point, a full-size bite is taken at a distance away from the first. This should make the suture appear to sit in a square configuration (Fig. 4.4a).

In tying this suture the tension has to be just right. If tied too loosely the skin edges fall apart, and if too tightly the skin edges pout too far and do not appose the skin edges. With the correct amount of tension the dermis and epidermis evert but still meet for accurate healing (Fig. 4.4b). This type of suture is of particular use in flexures, on the backs of hands and any site with loose skin, as it gives an excellent everting result.

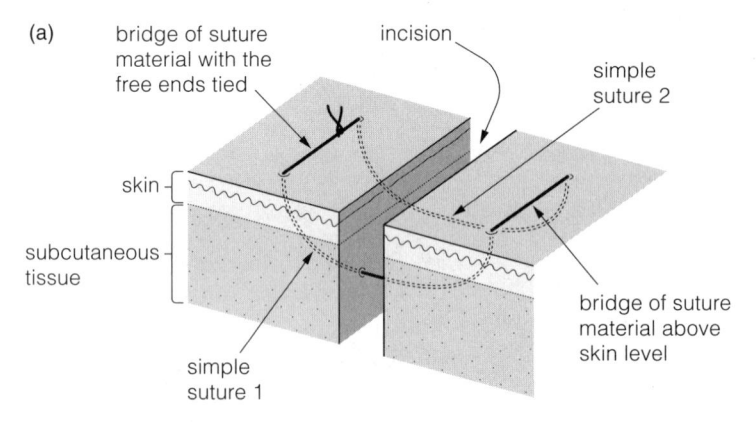

(a) bridge of suture material with the free ends tied — incision — simple suture 2 — skin — subcutaneous tissue — simple suture 1 — bridge of suture material above skin level

The horizontal mattress suture comprises two simple sutures and two bridges of suture material above the skin. In rough terms, the positioning of suture bites and suture bridges should approximate a square.

Fig. 4.4 *Horizontal mattress suture*

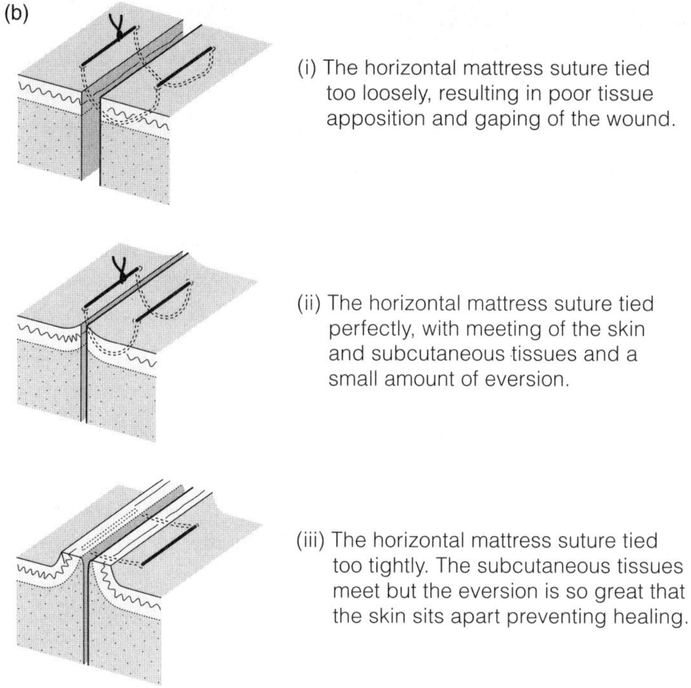

Basic Surgical Skills

(b)

(i) The horizontal mattress suture tied too loosely, resulting in poor tissue apposition and gaping of the wound.

(ii) The horizontal mattress suture tied perfectly, with meeting of the skin and subcutaneous tissues and a small amount of eversion.

(iii) The horizontal mattress suture tied too tightly. The subcutaneous tissues meet but the eversion is so great that the skin sits apart preventing healing.

Fig. 4.4 *Horizontal mattress suture (cont.)*

Continuous suture

Continuous, in this context, refers to the fact that there are no 'individual' sutures in this type of repair. The suture runs the entire length of the wound and is formed from a single piece of thread (Fig. 4.5). The suture is tied at the beginning of the wound and then the pattern (simple, vertical mattress or horizontal mattress) is followed until the end of the wound is reached and the suture is tied again. Apart from the previous variants, the simple suture may also be interlocked to improve the lie of the sutures. This does make the suture more ischaemic though. Continuous sutures are rarely used in modern practice.

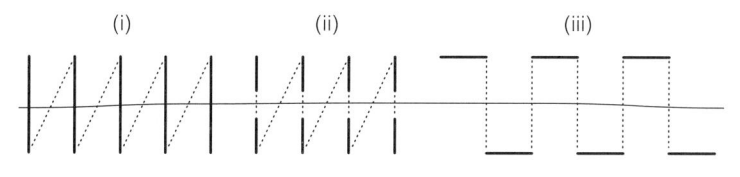

(i)   (ii)   (iii)

——— surface suture
·········· buried suture

(i) continuous simple suture
(ii) continuous vertical mattress suture
(iii) continuous horizontal mattress suture

Fig. 4.5 *Continuous suture—three versions*

Subcuticular suture

A subcuticular suture (Fig. 4.6) is an excellent way of closing skin without leaving unsightly cross-hatches in the scar. It is also far less ischaemic as the suture runs through the dermis (and therefore *in* the plane of the vessels) leading to reduced tissue pressure and ischaemia.

This suture is commenced by either burying a knot and bringing the suture up through the apex of the wound (absorbable threads) or by entering from the outside to the apex of the wound and securing the completed suture outside (Fig. 4.6a). Bites are taken parallel to the skin surface but through the dermis. Unless these bites are at the same depth an uneven vertical overlap will occur (Fig. 4.6b).

There are various theories on how much overlap should occur between suture bites, varying from none to almost 90%. If the suture has to be used for a long wound and it is to be removed, a *bridge* (loop of suture out onto the skin) may be used to allow for easier removal (Fig. 4.6c). The subcuticular suture technique may be performed with a nonabsorbable suture and removed, or an absorbable one and not removed.

If a nonabsorbable suture is used it may be tied to itself at the ends of the wound, or tied over the wound to create a loop (Fig. 4.6d). Beads and crimped steel have also been used to retain the ends. If an absorbable suture is used the end should be a buried knot. Commonly, in the past, straight needles have been used for this suture but in today's environment this should be discouraged and curved needles, in a needle holder, requested as a safer option.

Barron suture

The Barron suture (Fig. 4.7) is a special stitch that gives the advantages of both a horizontal mattress suture (eversion) and a subcuticular suture (low tissue ischaemia). It is used in situations where one side of the wound is likely to have poor blood supply and a normal suture may cause pressure ischaemia. Situations such as this occur when a flap of skin, with a narrow or distant base, needs to be secured in position.

The insertion starts as a simple suture but bites only as deep as the dermis. As it exits into the wound a subcuticular bite is taken (horizontally) for 5–10 mm. At the exit point the needle is once again used to complete a dermal-level, simple suture. It is then tied as a horizontal mattress (Fig. 4.7).

Basic Surgical Skills

(a) Starting the subcuticular suture (2 methods)

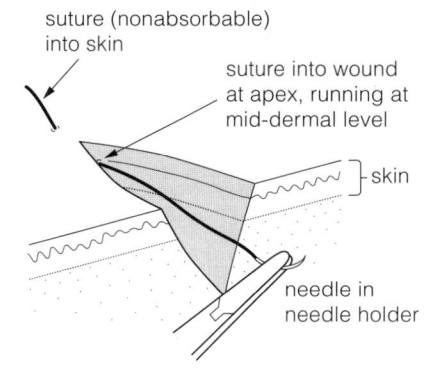

suture (nonabsorbable) into skin

suture into wound at apex, running at mid-dermal level

skin

needle in needle holder

(i) *The monofilament non-absorbable suture.* The suture is brought through the apex of the wound from outside, and is finished in the same way. It is secured by tying over the whole wound, knots at the end or crimping beads.

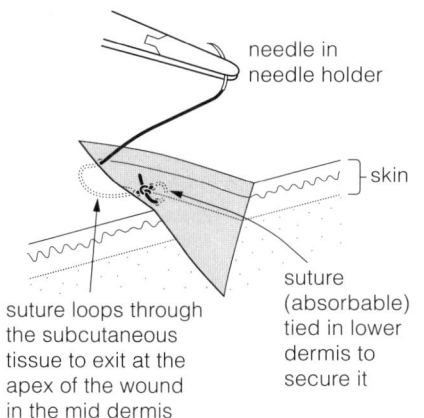

needle in needle holder

skin

suture loops through the subcutaneous tissue to exit at the apex of the wound in the mid dermis

suture (absorbable) tied in lower dermis to secure it

(ii) *The absorbable suture.* The suture is tied in the lower dermis or subcutaneous tissues to secure it. The thread is then looped through these tissues to exit at the apex of the wound at mid-dermal level.

(b) Subcuticular suture bite placement

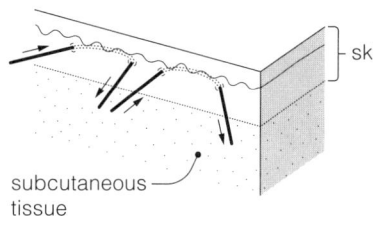

skin

subcutaneous tissue

(i) The subcuticular suture should enter and exit at approximately the junction of the upper and middle thirds of the dermis.

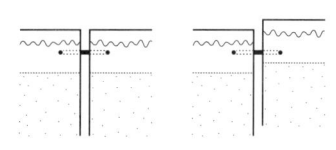

(ii) The picture on the left shows bites at the same dermal level, allowing even skin apposition. The picture on the right shows uneven bites at different dermal levels, causing uneven apposition and healing.

Fig. 4.6 *Subcuticular suture*

(c) Patterns of subcuticular stitch insertion

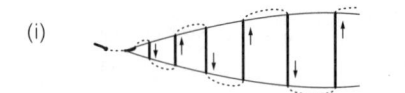

(i) Suture is inserted straight across from the exit point in the opposing dermis.

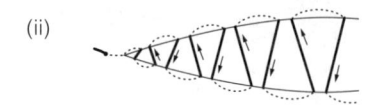

(ii) Suture is angled back towards the exit point of the last suture on the opposite side.

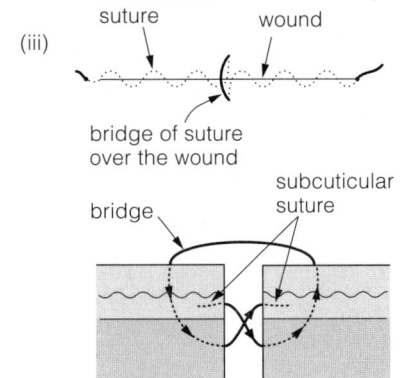

(iii) subcuticular suture / wound / bridge of suture over the wound / bridge / subcuticular suture

The bridge is inserted to ease removal. Once cut, this allows for two short sutures to be removed instead of one long one which may snap.

(d) Finishing a subcuticular suture (nonabsorbable)

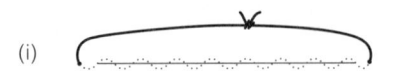

(i) Tied over the wound

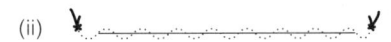

(ii) Tied to itself at the ends

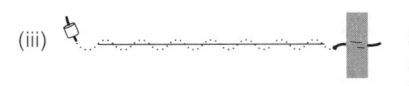

(iii) Secured with a crimped bead at one end and with a self-adhesive wound closure strip at the other

Fig. 4.6 *Subcuticular suture (cont.)*

Basic Surgical Skills

½ simple suture

½ simple suture

One side appears as a horizontal mattress suture and the other as a subcuticular suture.

dermal subcuticular component

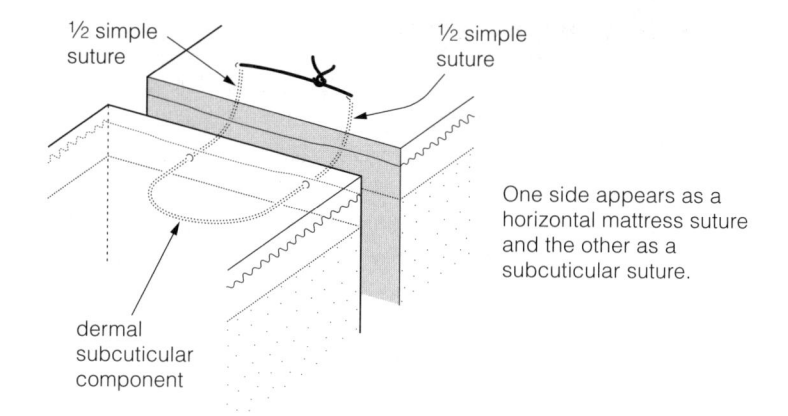

Fig. 4.7 *Barron suture*

Three-corner suture

In a similar vein to the Barron suture, the three-corner suture (Fig. 4.8) is a combination of horizontal mattress and subcuticular suture. It is used in stellate lacerations where three (or more) arms of the laceration come together. In the 'flattest' of the surfaces a simple suture is begun but inserted only as deep as the low dermis. The subcuticular part of the suture is then carried through the dermis at the apices of the other tissue components. To complete the suture, a dermal-depth simple suture bite is inserted parallel to the first part of the suture and the two ends tied (Fig. 4.8).

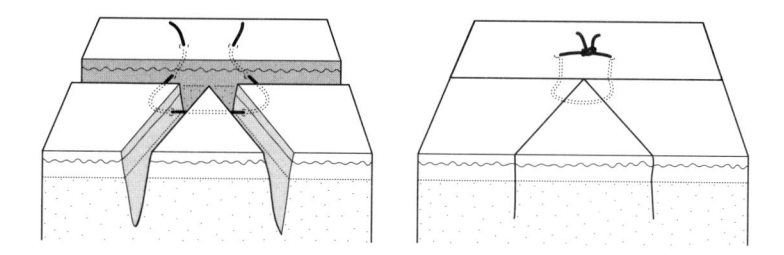

A variant of the Barron suture, the three-corner suture is used to hold the apices of stellate lacerations. The illustration on the right shows how it appears when tied.

Fig. 4.8 *Three-corner suture*

Surgical knot tying

The ability to tie secure 'knots' rapidly, in any situation or body cavity, is an essential part of surgical practice. The actions with which to do this must be extremely familiar for the occasional operator and pure reflex for a surgeon. The life of a patient may depend on the security of one ligature at a virtually inaccessible point. Slippage of a tie like this may result in death from exsanguination or potentially major morbidity from the blood loss and its haemodynamic sequelae.

Principles of knot tying

The formation of a knot in a suture can be described as the 'intertwining of threads for the purpose of joining them' (Kirk 1995). What we call a knot, however, is strictly a *bend* or *hitch* as the definition of knot is 'a knob or node' in the arboreal (tree) sense. The security of any tied suture is improved by the use of certain patterns of knot and the friction between threads. This friction factor is affected by the size of contact area between threads, the tightness of tying, and the suture material that is used. Unfortunately, kinking of the thread or inadequate tightening can reduce knot security by either slippage or breakage.

A *reef knot* is the basic pattern from which all surgical knots derive. This may have two turns of the thread, as opposed to the standard single turn, and be called a *surgeon's knot*. The main advantage of this pattern is the greater friction between threads, leading to improved security of the first throw.

The basic element of the reef knot is a *half-hitch*. This manoeuvre is where one thread is looped around the other. To complete the knot a mirror image of the first throw is performed. If the reverse throw is performed a *granny knot* is formed (Fig. 4.9).

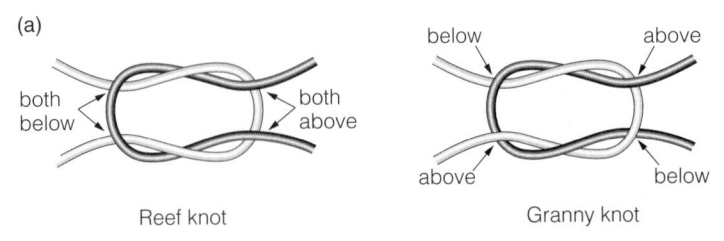

(a)

Reef knot — both below, both above

Granny knot — below, above, above, below

When tying a reef knot, note how the two free ends of one suture emerge from either above or below the loop created by the other suture. In a granny knot the free ends emerge one above and one below each loop.

Fig. 4.9a *Reef knot versus granny knot*

(b)

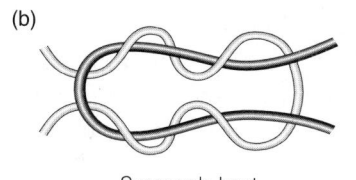

The surgeon's knot follows the same pattern as the reef knot except there are two throws on each side of the knot instead of one.

Surgeon's knot

Fig. 4.9b *Surgeon's knot*

To ensure correct orientation and good security of the knot the ends of the thread should be pulled at 180° to each other. This will 'lay down' the knot as flat as possible and prevent the thread pulling into a *sliding hitch* (Fig. 4.10). Depending on the suture material, up to four throws may be required for a standard knot and as many as eight in certain situations.

The next two sections deal with two different ways of tying the same knot. The first, and probably simplest to learn, is the instrument-tied reef knot. The second is a one-handed technique for tying reef knots. A two-handed technique is the third common method of tying a reef knot but this will only be discussed, not described. Both descriptions are for right-handed operators. Left-handed surgeons should substitute the words *right* and *left* for each other and do similarly for *clockwise* and *anti-clockwise*.

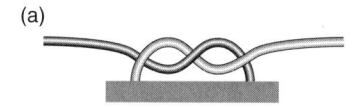

(a)

By pulling the ends of a suture at 180° the half-hitch will sit flat against the tissue surface.

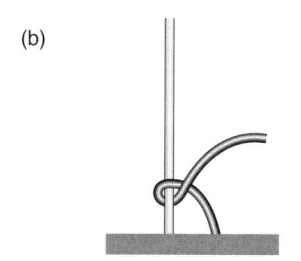

(b)

If the two threads are pulled at 90° one tends to loop around the other and slide—hence the term 'sliding hitch'. A row of these will potentially allow the suture to slip, come loose and unravel.

Fig. 4.10 *Flat 'laid-down' knot versus sliding half-hitch*

Instrument knot

Trying a reef knot with an instrument is probably the commonest method of tying sutures in the skin and subcutaneous tissues. Hand tying can be used but takes significantly more thread to accomplish and so is less economical.

Step 1

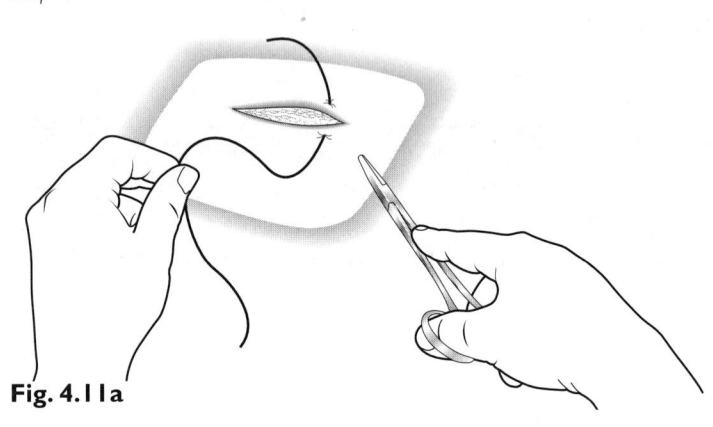

Fig. 4.11a

Insert the suture and pull it through so that there is a long end which still has the needle attached and a short end on the other side of the wound. Convention would usually have the long end on the side of the wound closest to you (Fig. 4.11a).

Step 2

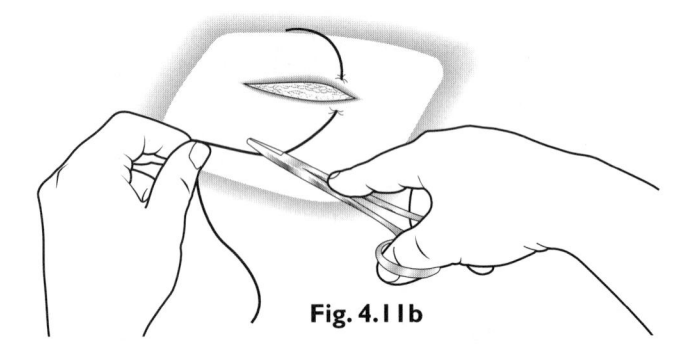

Fig. 4.11b

'Palm', or put down, your forceps and hold the long end of the suture in the left hand. Pull it vertically upwards to straighten (but not put tension on) the thread. At the same time, with needle holders held in the right hand, play a tennis forehand shot towards the straightened thread (Fig. 4.11b).

Basic Surgical Skills

Step 3

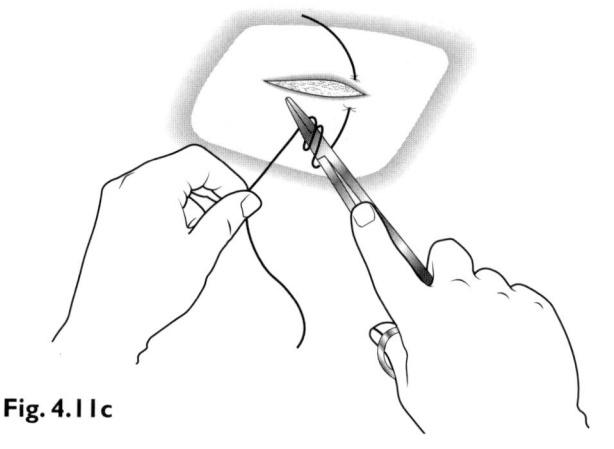

Fig. 4.11c

When the needle holder makes contact, the long end of the thread is wound over and around the jaws of the needle holder, in a clockwise spiral, and back around to the vertical. This may be done twice to create the double loop of a surgeon's knot. Once completed, the tip of the short thread end should be grasped (Fig. 4.11c).

Step 4

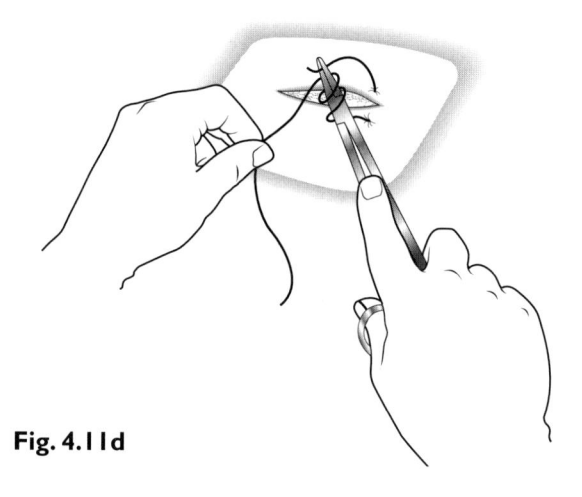

Fig. 4.11d

The short end of the thread is drawn towards the opposite side of the wound from which it originally lay, through the loops of thread wound around the needle holder. The long thread end, in turn, is pushed in the opposite direction (Fig. 4.11d).

Step 5

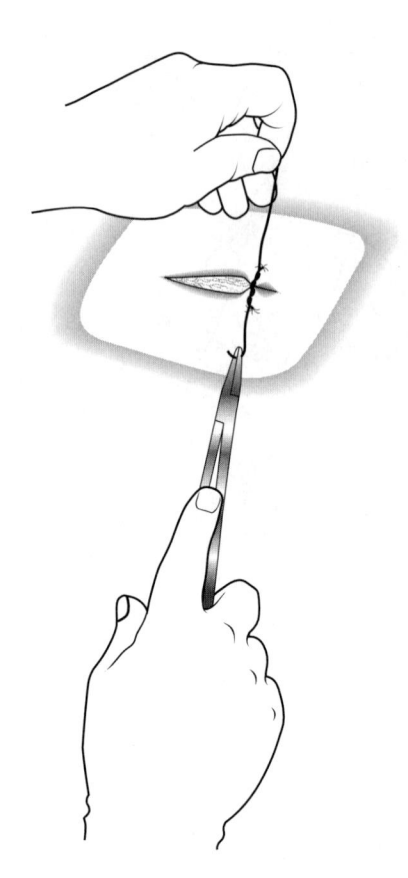

Fig. 4.11e

The knot is tightened by continuing to pull in the same directions, with the ends of the threads held at 180° to each other and in the line of the inserted suture (Fig. 4.11e).

Step 6

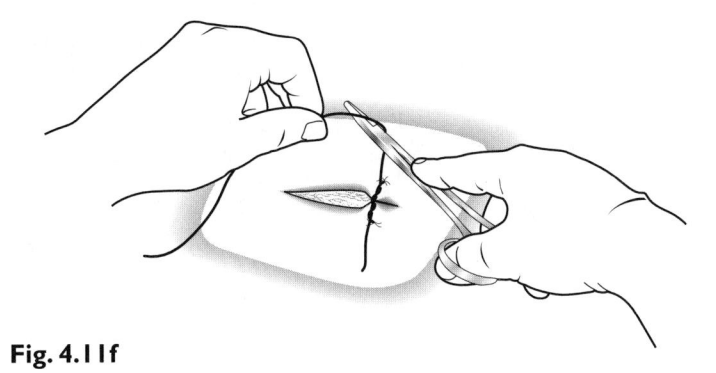

Fig. 4.11f

Once again pull the long end of the thread vertically with the left hand. Ensure that this is not done so hard as to loosen the tightened first throw or to convert it into a hitch. With the needle holders still held in the right hand, play a tennis backhand shot towards the straightened thread (Fig. 4.11f).

Step 7

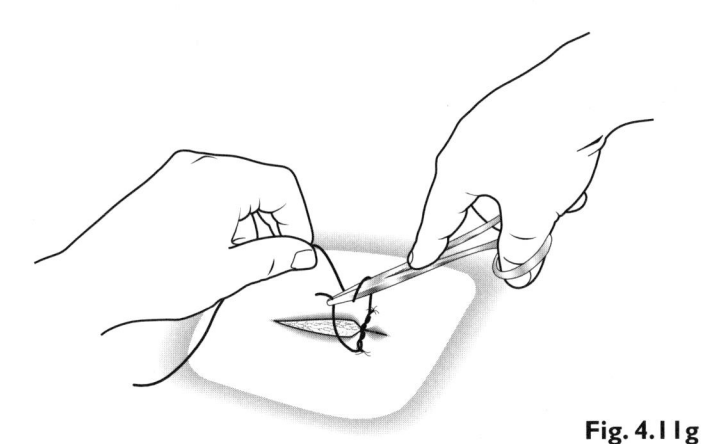

Fig. 4.11g

When the needle holder contacts the thread, wind the thread over and around the jaws of the needle holder in an anti-clockwise spiral over the instrument and back around to the vertical. Once again, this may be done twice to create the double loop of a surgeon's knot. Once completed, the tip of the short thread end should again be grasped (Fig. 4.11g).

Step 8

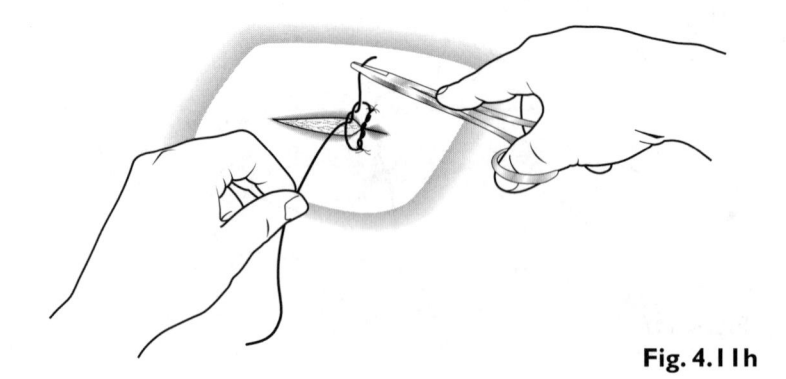

Fig. 4.11h

Once again grasp the short end of the thread and draw it in the opposite direction from the first throw, through the loops of thread around the needle holder. Tighten the knot by pulling the ends at 180° to each other. This completes the reef or surgeon's knot (Fig. 4.11h).

Step 9

Repeat steps 2 to 8 as required, producing the appropriate number of throws to secure the suture.

One-handed knot

While called a one-handed knot, two hands are required to tie it. The 'one-handed' title comes from the fact that the second hand is merely an anchor for one of the threads, all throws of the knot being generated by the fingers of one hand only. Both hands are also required to secure the knot down snugly.

This description is for right-handers, as the left hand is used for tying. This means that an instrument in the right hand (usually a needle holder with needle) does not have to be placed down on the patient while tying the knot. Instead it may be palmed while the right hand anchors the long end of the thread. This description also assumes that the short (tag) end of the thread is away from you and the long (needle) end is closer (Fig. 4.12a).

There are two distinct phases to tying this knot. Phase one generates the first throw of the knot and is demonstrated by steps 1–8. The second throw is described in steps 9–13.

Step 1

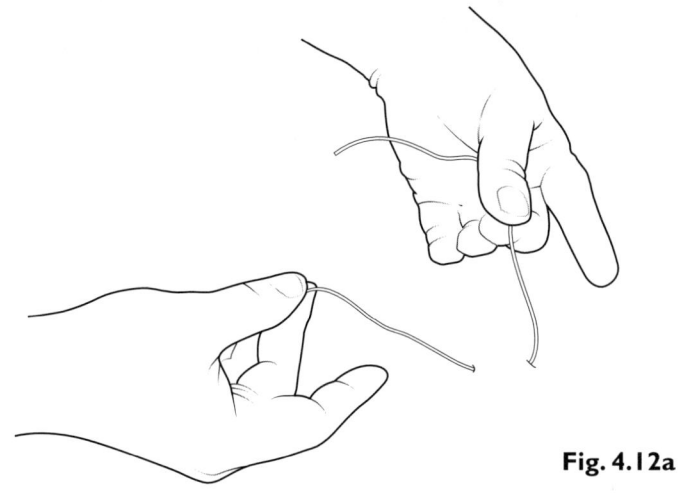

Fig. 4.12a

Both ends of the thread are grasped in an 'underhand pinch' grip between the thumb and middle fingers of both hands. Both forearms should be in the mid-prone position (Fig. 4.12a).

Step 2

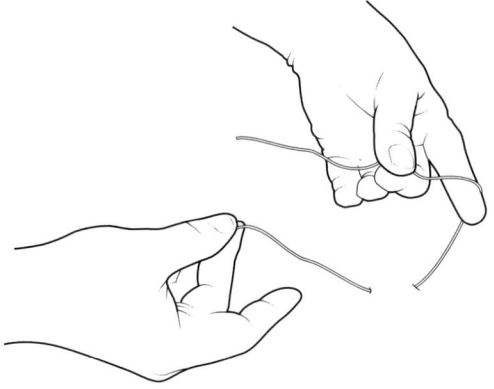

Fig. 4.12b

The left index finger is placed *under* the thread held by the left hand and over the thread held by the right hand (Fig. 4.12b).

Step 3

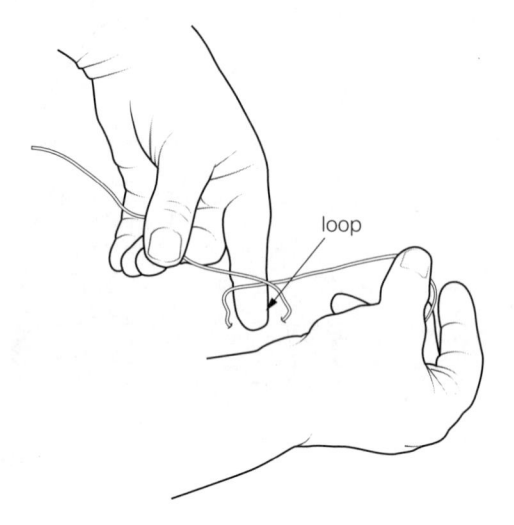

Fig. 4.12c

The right hand is then pushed forwards, drawing the thread over the index finger, and the two threads form a loop (Fig. 4.12c).

Step 4

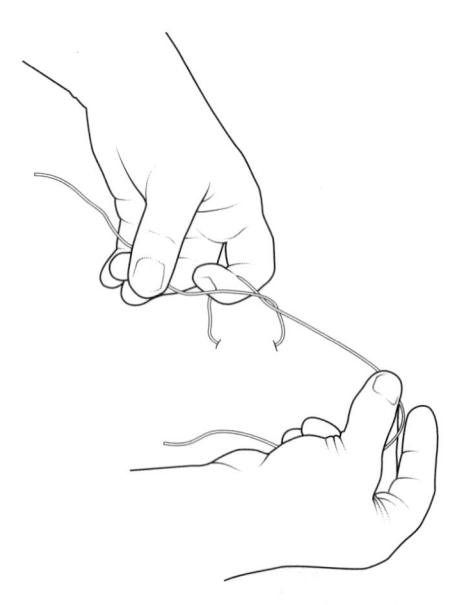

Fig. 4.12d

The left index finger is flexed (curled up) so that it lies below the left hand's thread but at the same time traps the right hand's thread in the flexed distal interphalangeal joint (Fig. 4.12d).

Basic Surgical Skills

Step 5

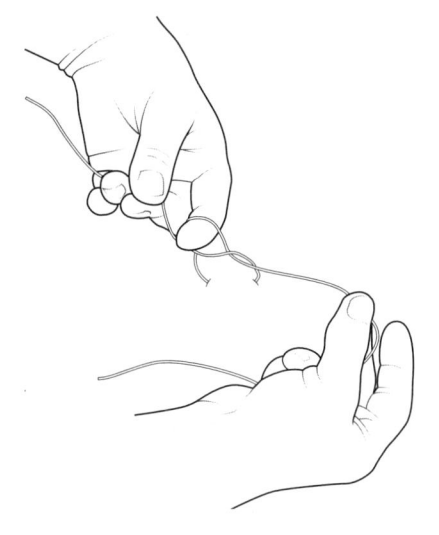

Fig. 4.12e

Extension of the interphalangeal joints of the left index finger, while the metacarpophalangeal (knuckle) joint is still flexed, will pick up the left hand's thread in preparation to use the back of the finger to sweep it through the loop mentioned in step 3 (Fig. 4.12e).

Step 6

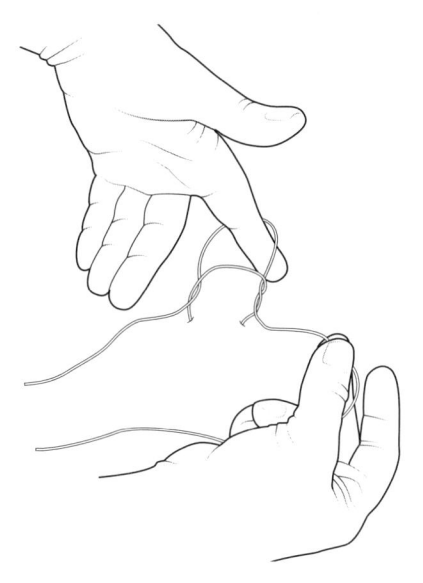

Fig. 4.12f

Full extension of the metacarpophalangeal (knuckle) joint of the left index finger is combined with extension of the wrist, and at the same time the left-hand thread is released. This manoeuvre will draw the left-hand thread through the loop (Fig. 4.12f).

Step 7

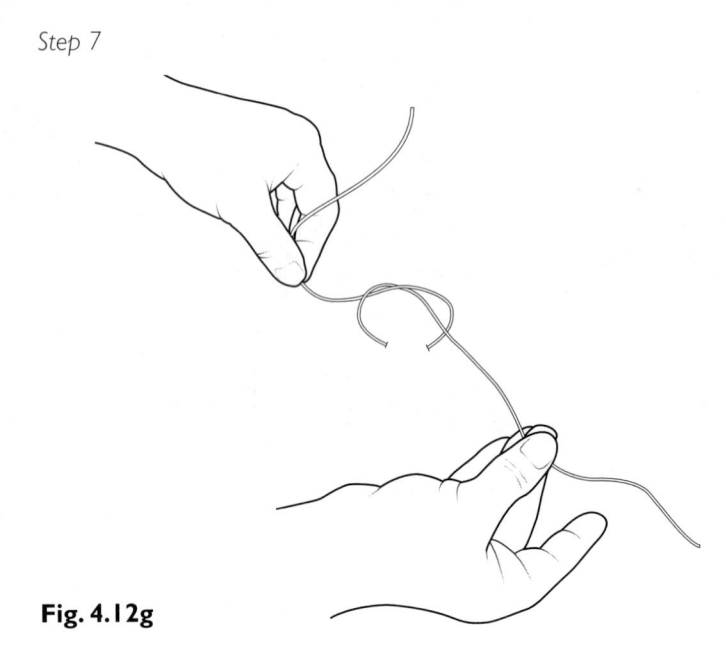

Fig. 4.12g

The left-hand thread is then re-grasped in an 'overhand pinch' grip between the thumb and index finger of the left hand with the left forearm fully pronated (Fig. 4.12g).

Step 8

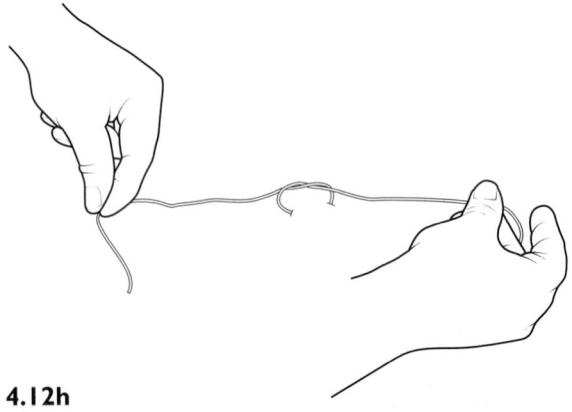

Fig. 4.12h

The throw is then laid down by bringing the left hand towards the operator and pushing the right hand (still in its original orientation) directly away from the operator. This should be done with the threads at 180° and will result in the first half of the reef knot lying flat against the tissues (Fig. 4.12h).

Step 9

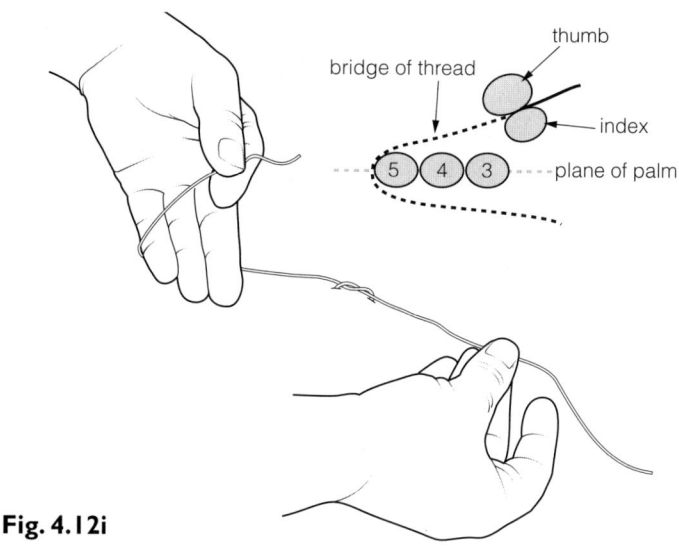

Fig. 4.12i

Next, fully supinate the left forearm with the thread still held between the thumb and index finger but with these two fingers above the plane of the palm. The left-hand thread should now run down and towards the operator, around the little finger or ulnar side of the hand, and back to the wound, creating a *bridge* (Fig. 4.12i).

Step 10

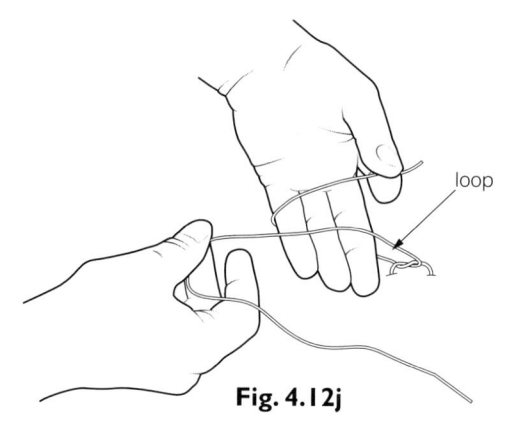

Fig. 4.12j

The right-hand thread must now be brought back towards the operator and laid flat on the three outstretched fingers of the left hand at the level of the PIP joint. The right hand should now be closer to the operator than the left hand. This also creates a loop of thread behind the left hand (Fig. 4.12j).

Step 11

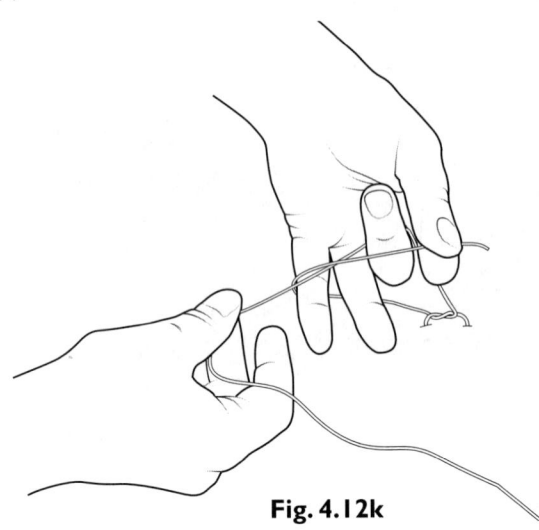

Fig. 4.12k

The middle finger of the left hand is flexed over the thread lying flat on the palm and positioned underneath the *bridged* left-hand thread (Fig. 4.12k).

Step 12

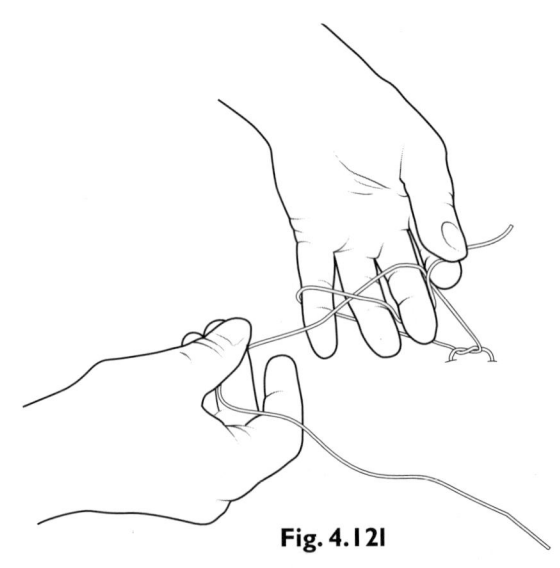

Fig. 4.12l

Extension of the left middle finger will pick up the thread (Fig. 4.12l) and extension of the wrist will pull the thread through the loop described in step 10 (Fig. 4.12m).

Basic Surgical Skills

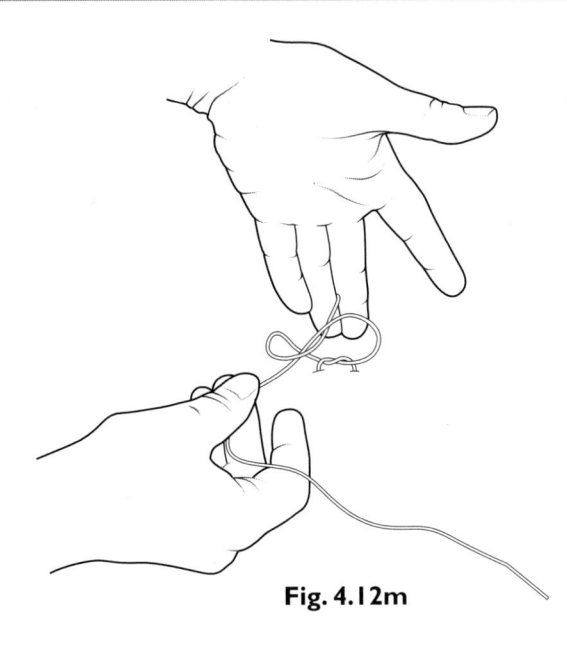

Fig. 4.12m

Step 13

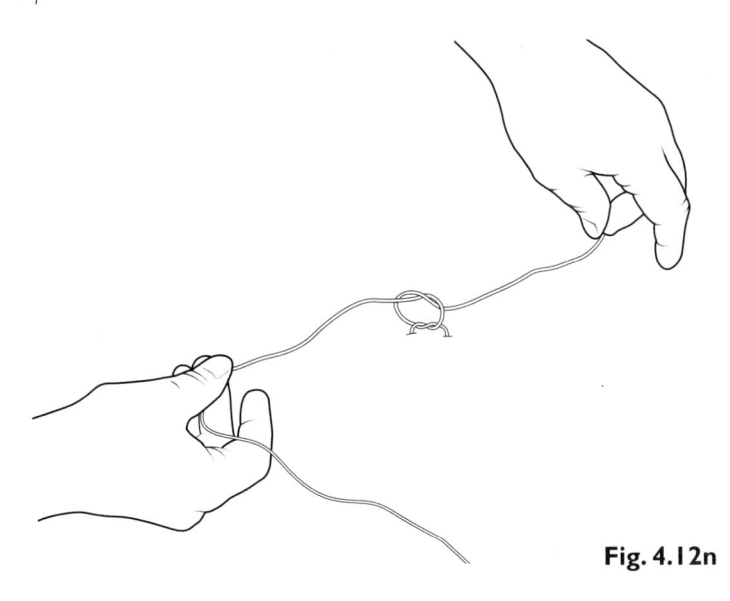

Fig. 4.12n

The left-hand thread must now be firmly grasped between the thumb and middle finger of the left hand. This hand is pushed away from, and the right hand brought towards, the operator with the threads at 180°. This will lay the second throw of the reef knot flatly against the tissues (Fig. 4.12n).

Step 14

Repeat steps 1 to 13 to create a double reef knot. As an added feature, two throws of the thread can be brought through the loops in steps 6 and 12 to create a surgeon's knot.

Two-handed knot

The two-handed method of tying a reef knot is most useful when wishing to maintain strict tension on both threads. This may apply if tying down a deep hole or if the structure is difficult to secure and must be kept compressed while tying. It is mostly used by gynaecologists during hysterectomy to secure the ovarian vascular pedicles but is sometimes employed by other groups of surgeons (such as general or thoracic surgeons), also when tying large vascular pedicles. It is important that all surgeons are competent in this technique but is less relevant for the junior trainee or occasional minor proceduralist.

Basic surgical techniques

Many special skills are required to perform surgical procedures safely. While some of these skills are unique to a single specialty the great majority are used across all specialties. This section deals with many skills common to virtually every branch of surgery.

Incisions and excisions

A scalpel is the instrument traditionally used to incise skin (a basic introduction to the use of a scalpel is found in Chapter 2).

The scalpel should always be held so that the blade is at 90° to the skin surface. This will ensure a neat vertical cut that will heal with the least scarring. There are two common methods of holding a scalpel (see Chap. 2)—the *underhand grip* and the *pen grip* (Fig. 4.13a, b). The underhand grip is used for larger, straight, sweeping incisions and the pen grip for finer, curved work and sharp dissection.

Smaller or curved incisions are often marked to ensure accuracy of placement, or adequacy of margins (e.g. skin lesion or mastectomy). Sometimes these marks are cross-hatched to ensure accuracy of closure (e.g. thoracotomy or thyroidectomy). This marking must withstand removal when the skin is prepared and so should be made with a permanent marker. Red ink, or a degradable pigment, should be used to reduce the risk of this mark tattooing the skin if pigment is drawn down into the dermis during the incision.

Basic Surgical Skills

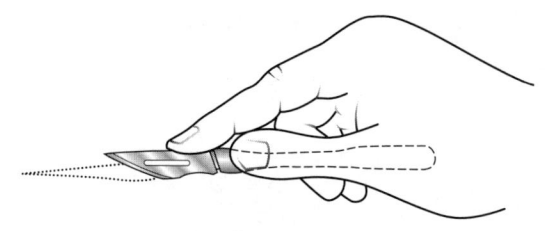

(a) The underhand or table-knife grip, used for long incisions.

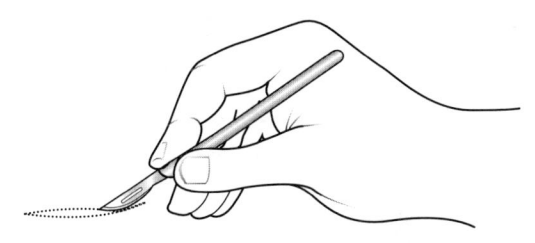

(b) The pen grip is used for fine incisions or excisions and for dissection with the scalpel.

Fig 4.13 *Holding a scalpel*

For the best effect the whole length of the blade, not just the tip, should be employed in cutting. In a long skin incision, such as that for a laparotomy, a larger handle and blade (e.g. size 4 handle and 22 blade) are required. Held in the *underhand grip* (Fig. 4.13a), like a dinner knife, the depth of cut is controlled by a combination of smoothly drawing the blade over the tissues and applying constant firm pressure with the forearm. With experience this can be controlled with great accuracy.

The traditional approach is to make the majority of larger incisions with a scalpel, and this certainly still holds in emergency situations. Given modern concerns about sharps, it is now quite common to use the scalpel to divide only the epidermis and most, or all, of the dermis. From here the diathermy is used to complete the incision to the desired depth.

For the finer and more precise incisions required in the excision of small skin lesions, the debridement of dirty wound edges and many plastic surgery procedures, a small handle and blade should be used (e.g. size 3 handle and 15 blade). This scalpel should be held in the *pen grip* (Fig. 4.13b) and most of the movement imparted on the blade comes from the hand and fingers. With this grip the surgeon's wrist can also be placed against the patient, an instrument or their other hand to steady the blade while cutting. The full length of the blade should still be used for the incision, and diathermy is sometimes used to complete it.

Let us illustrate the finer of these two techniques with excision of a skin lesion as the example.

Step 1

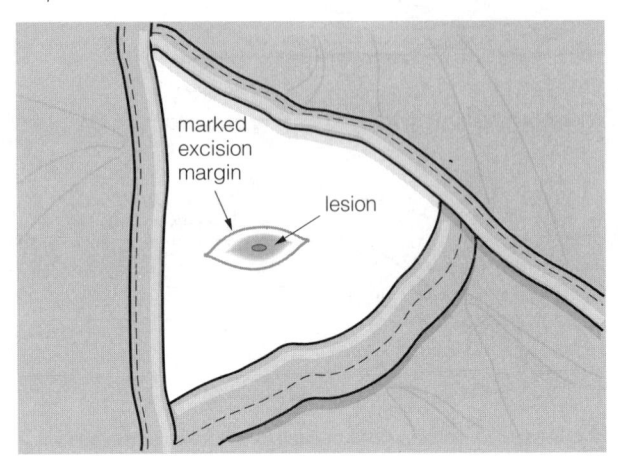

Fig. 4.14a

An ellipse should be marked around the lesion to ensure adequate margins of excision and to ensure that the planned incision is constructed in the best possible line for closure (Fig. 4.14a).

Step 2

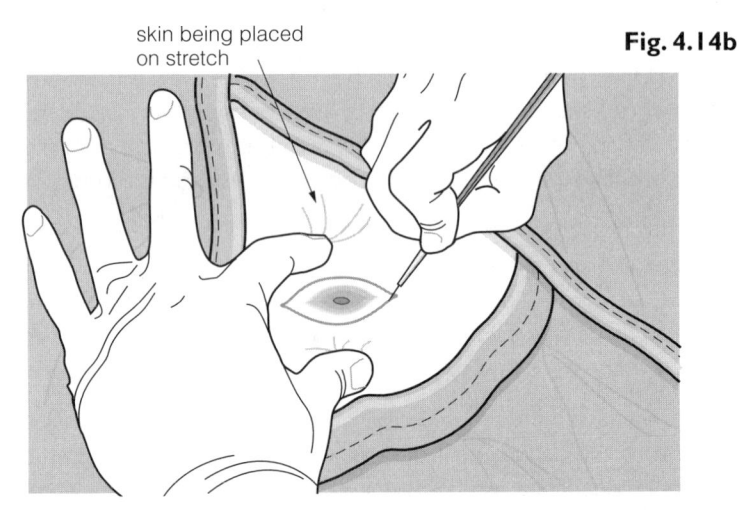

Fig. 4.14b

In making the first incision the scalpel, held in a *pen grip* (Fig. 4.13b) with the blade vertical, is drawn along the more *dependent* of the two marked lines. This tactic prevents blood from running over, and obscuring, tissues that have not yet been incised. The skin to be incised should be placed on stretch with the other hand, preferably at right angles to the line of incision (Fig. 4.14b).

Step 3

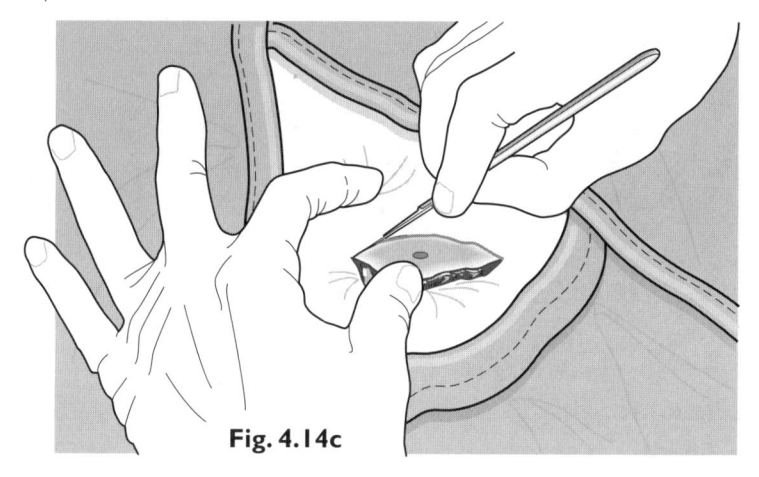

Fig. 4.14c

Once the scalpel blade is through dermis of the 'lower' margin, the upper incision can be made. A tissue forcep may need to be placed on the already cut edge to assist in providing tension to cut against (Fig. 4.14c).

Step 4

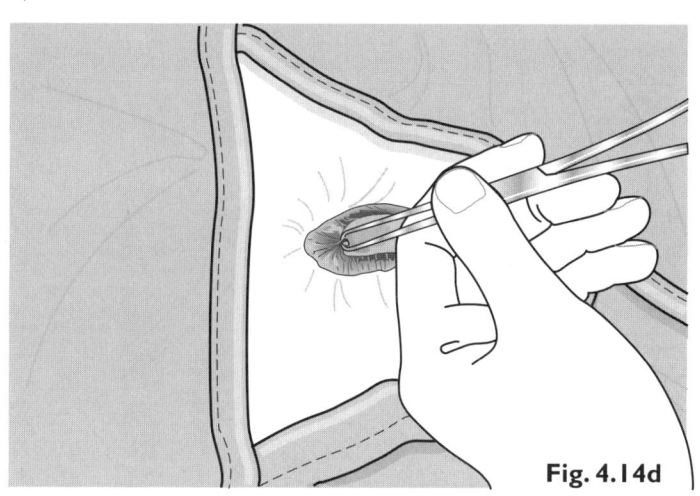

Fig. 4.14d

Particular attention must be paid to completely incising one angled corner of the specimen. This can then be lifted with tissue forceps and the subcutaneous tissue (fat) dissected by knife, scissor or diathermy down to, and along, the plane of the deep fascia. This dissection should proceed almost vertically to its deepest extent as a shelving (V) incision may leave behind involved tissue (Fig. 4.14d).

Step 5

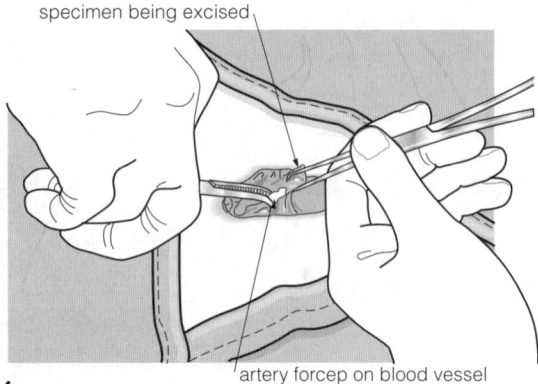

Fig. 4.14e

During dissection of the specimen (step 4), or after complete removal of the specimen, haemostasis must be obtained. Diathermy or ligation are the commonest methods, although twisting vessels and pressure are also valid techniques (Fig. 4.14e).

Step 6

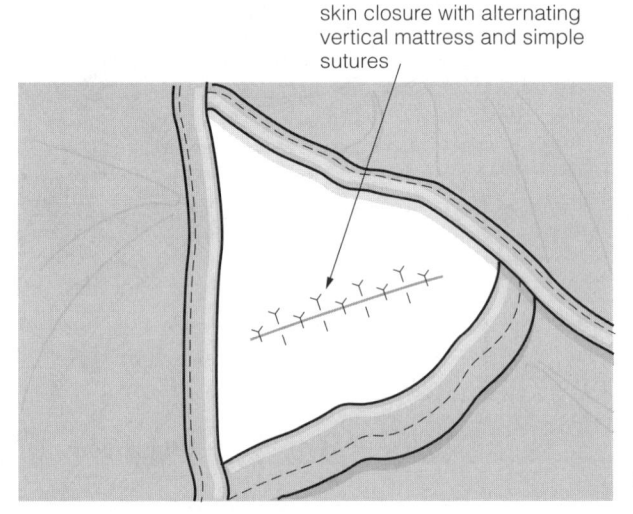

Fig. 4.14f

Closure is now effected using a combination of deep (if required) and cutaneous sutures.

In contrast to the above procedure, a mid-line abdominal, laparotomy incision is made by cutting down through all layers of the abdominal wall to the peritoneum. A combination of scalpel, diathermy and (sometimes) scissors are used for this task. The initial cut should be carried through the epidermis and dermis in one long sweeping motion of the whole blade (not just the tip) held in the *underhand grip* (Fig. 4.13a) which may be practised in the air over the abdomen prior to commencing. Once through skin, the fat and linea alba may be cut with scalpel, scissors or diathermy. Peritoneum is then lifted between two artery forceps and nicked with a scalpel blade. This allows viscera to fall away from the anterior abdominal wall with the in-rush of air. Remnant tissue can then be cut with heavy scissors or diathermy.

In concluding this section it is probably wise to reflect upon the ease with which a scalpel cuts. It is razor sharp and will cut anything it is brought against under pressure or tension. This property makes the scalpel a potentially dangerous tool that can easily incise or divide a vital structure (e.g. peripheral nerve or vessel) inadvertently if appropriate care is not taken. This risk also applies to any body parts of the scrub team that the scalpel comes in contact with!

Following the simple rules below (which are also contained in the instrument chapter) will minimise this risk.

1. Do not cut anything that cannot actually be seen.
2. If the tissue to be divided is superficial to a vital structure, insert an instrument or cutting guide between them.
3. If dissecting near a known structure (e.g. nerve or vessel), cut in the line of the structure to prevent dividing it accidentally. This does not prevent incising it longitudinally but these injuries are usually much less serious.
4. Plan (and mark) your incisions and practise the cut in the air first.
5. If cutting in a deep cavity, time spent improving the access and exposure equates to time saved repairing a potential error.
6. There is no substitute for excellent sharps technique in the prevention of penetrating wounds in the operator and scrub team.

Debridement

Debridement is a term applied to the manual removal of foreign, dead, devitalised and contaminated materials from an open wound (Fig. 4.15). This procedure reduces the chance of infection by the elimination of foreign bodies and ischaemic areas of dead tissue as well as

Basic Surgical Skills

(a)

scrubbing brush

irrigation solution

shaver

shaved area

bowl

When preparing a wound for debridement it needs a gross cleansing first. This is done following anaesthesia. Shaving, irrigation and the removal of grease, dirt and gross contamination with a scrubbing brush are the first steps in the process of wound repair.

(b)

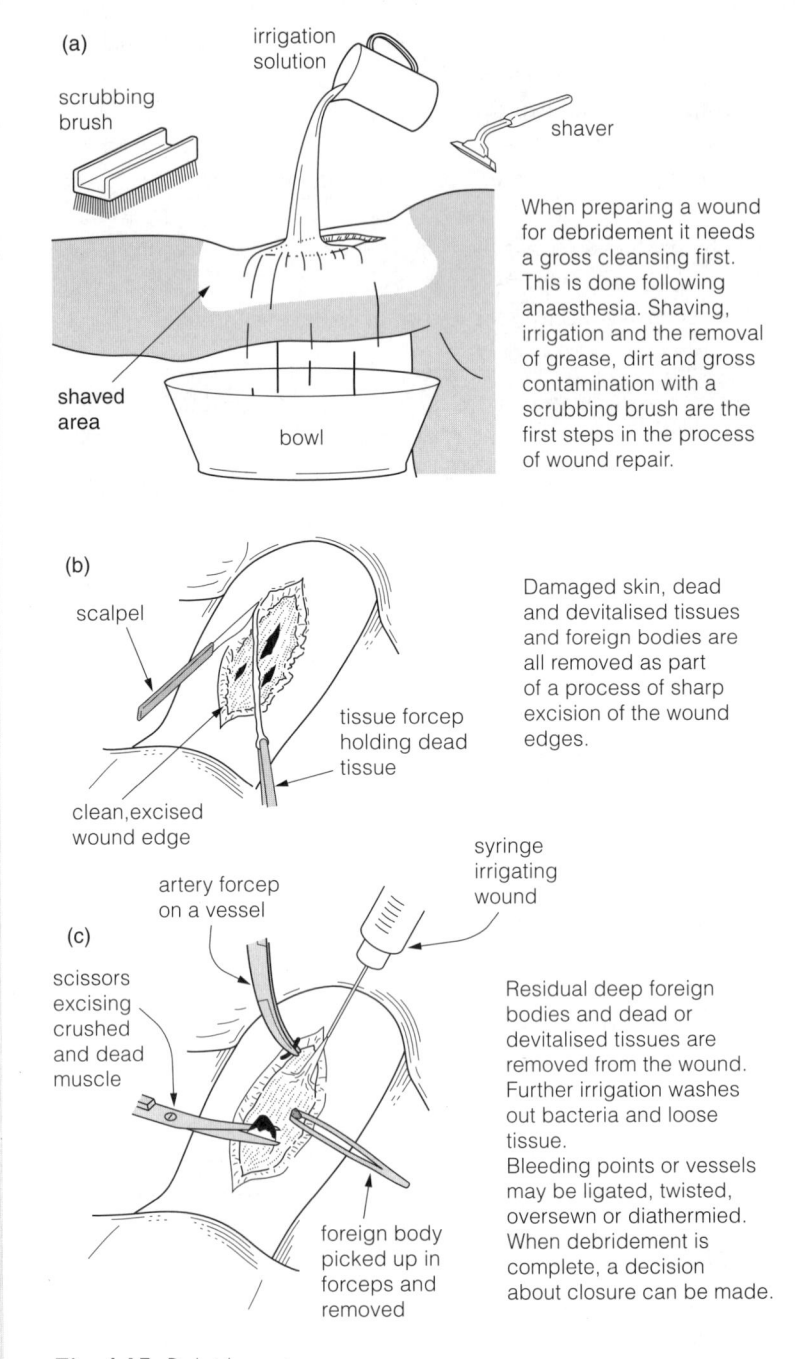

scalpel

tissue forcep holding dead tissue

clean, excised wound edge

Damaged skin, dead and devitalised tissues and foreign bodies are all removed as part of a process of sharp excision of the wound edges.

(c)

scissors excising crushed and dead muscle

artery forcep on a vessel

syringe irrigating wound

foreign body picked up in forceps and removed

Residual deep foreign bodies and dead or devitalised tissues are removed from the wound. Further irrigation washes out bacteria and loose tissue.
Bleeding points or vessels may be ligated, twisted, oversewn or diathermied. When debridement is complete, a decision about closure can be made.

Fig. 4.15 *Debridement*

reducing the amount of any bacterial contamination present. The debridement process may be as simple as irrigating a minor wound with saline or may require general anaesthesia and extensive removal of tissues. No matter where the wound is situated, the object of the exercise is to minimise infective complications by converting a dirty or contaminated wound into a surgically clean one. The ultimate extension of this concept is the en-bloc excision of an entire contaminated wound to leave a fresh surgically created wound, with no contamination, ready for primary closure!

There is no single defined way in which to debride a wound or any prescribed number of debridements required to declare a wound clean or fit for closure. The broad aim is to remove any material that may impair healing. At the time of initial debridement any tissue of uncertain viability may be left to declare itself and a second or even third toilet procedure planned to complete the process. In general, skin is pink, fat yellow, fascia white/silver and muscle red/pink. Any tissues of abnormal colour should be suspected of being dubiously viable or dead. Principles, therefore, must be followed to ensure consistent success in a variety of situations.

Steps in wound debridement

1. The wound should initially be irrigated and scrubbed to remove surface debris and this is often done once the patient is anaesthetised but prior to prepping and draping.
2. The site is then widely prepped and draped. Tourniquets should be avoided except in the presence of major vascular trauma—they obscure the presence of bleeding that confirms tissue viability but which needs to be controlled prior to closure.
3. All foreign bodies and dead tissue must be removed or excised.
4. Crushed or dubiously viable tissue must be fully excised if primary closure is planned; or it may be left to declare itself if second-look debridement and delayed primary closure or secondary healing are planned.
5. The skin edges and deep surfaces should be cut back to bleeding tissue. This gives the double benefit of ensuring viability and providing vertical skin edges for a fine scar. A scalpel should be used to debride skin and this, or scissors, may also be used for soft tissues. The process involves a gradual trimming of tissues back to a clean and bleeding edge. It is important when cutting skin edges to provide good counter-traction so that only a fine sliver of damaged

tissue is removed. Care should be taken to debride in the line of any longitudinal structures (e.g. limb arteries, veins or nerves) to avoid transection or damage. In small wounds a complete (en-bloc) excision of the entire lesion will provide surgically clean tissue for primary closure.

6. Further irrigation is used to wash out bacteria, residual foreign bodies and small non-viable tissue fragments. Irrigation is usually in the form of normal saline. Betadine solutions, antibiotics and other antiseptics are occasionally used but there is little evidence of their benefit. In fact, there is research evidence to suggest that these may all cause damage at a cellular level that impairs the healing process. The irrigant may be poured or squirted onto the wound and is usually caught in a kidney dish or gallipot to minimise spillage and mess. In small wounds a 10 ml syringe and 23# needle deliver irrigant at a near perfect pressure, when squeezed gently.

7. Adequate haemostasis is essential prior to completing the debridement but, especially if the wound is to be primarily closed, excessive diathermy or ligation can leave dead tissues with foreign (suture) material as foci for infection.

8. Once completed, the decision as to whether a second-look debridement is required must be made and the appropriate mode of closure attended to. A small Penrose-type drain may help drain haematoma, seroma and pus from the wound if primary closure is attempted.

Table 4.1 Principles of traumatic wound debridement

1. Pre-op irrigation and scrubbing to remove surface debris
2. Wide prepping and draping
3. Avoid tourniquets unless vital
4. Excise all foreign bodies and dead tissue
5. Excise crushed or dubiously viable tissue if primary closure is planned or leave it to declare and plan a second-look debridement
6. Cut skin edges and deep surfaces back to bleeding tissue. Debride in the line of any longitudinal structures (e.g. limb arteries, veins or nerves) to avoid transection or damage
7. Further irrigate the wound to wash out bacteria, residual foreign bodies and small non-viable tissue fragments. Use normal saline, not povidone-iodine solution, antibiotics or other antiseptics as they may be tissue-toxic
8. Obtain haemostasis prior to completing the debridement
9. Decide whether a second-look debridement or formal closure is required

Debridement is a vital part of managing all traumatic or infected wounds. It has only a small role to play in major elective surgery but it is an essential skill required by all surgeons who treat wounds.

Haemostasis and diathermy

Principles

Bleeding has the dual problem of being a threat to the operation's success by blood obscuring the operative field, or clot promoting postoperative infection, and to the patient's well-being with the potential problems of operation failure, haematoma, infections and even exsanguination. The prevention or reduction of bleeding from the operative site is known as haemostasis. There are two main principles in the process of haemostasis. The first is the *prevention of bleeding* and the second the *management of bleeding*.

While these processes may sound straightforward there are other factors such as experience, knowledge of techniques and calmness in difficult situations which affect the potential outcome of haemostasis. The prevention and management of bleeding, then, relies not only on good technique but also on good clinical judgment; and both of these are especially important in the handling of acute torrential bleeding.

Prevention of bleeding

Prevention of bleeding and its consequences begins *preoperatively* with the correction of anaemia and detection of clotting disorders. During the *intraoperative* phase the use of gentle and appropriate techniques of dissection and exposure will reduce bleeding. Coupled with this, a strong anatomical knowledge will prevent inadvertent damage to major vascular structures.

Preoperative strategies

Coagulopathy should be actively sought in the at-risk patient (e.g. jaundice, liver disease, uraemia or anticoagulants). This should be corrected with Vitamin K (if related to hepatic causes) and/or clotting factor rich solutions, such as FFP or cryoprecipitate. Vitamin K should be commenced as early as possible during the clinical course on any jaundiced patients who may require surgery and in all jaundiced patients with deranged clotting. Intravenous clotting solutions should be started in the immediate preoperative period, to maximise their efficacy, or commenced during the procedure if not obtainable before this.

Platelets are rarely of use in the thrombocytopenic patient. They do not become active for some hours and normal clotting can still occur with platelet counts of as low as 40 ($\times 10^6$ per mm^3). If a patient is found to be thrombocytopenic the correct course is to investigate this and find, then treat, the underlying cause.

Oral anticoagulants are another common cause of deranged clotting. Aspirin should be ceased at least one week prior to operating and warfarin approximately 4–5 days prior. An INR check the day before surgery will confirm that clotting has returned to normal levels. If there is a pressing reason to remain on anticoagulants, either surgery should be delayed until they can be stopped or the patient managed with heparin in the perioperative period. This allows closer titration of anticoagulation, easy reversal and the ability to use a rapidly acting antidote (protamine sulphate) if required.

Preparation of a preoperative cross-match (or group and hold serum) will facilitate the provision of blood should the need arise. Local haemorrhage may also be reduced by the use of a pre-incision injection of vasoconstrictors and tourniquets on limbs.

Intraoperative strategies

Careful incision of the skin with the use of diathermy to cut subcutaneous tissue will result in the coagulation of all but the larger vessels. Any bleeding vessels may then be grasped and diathermied. Alternatively, the use of accurate dissection with the application of artery forceps and vessels ligation is equally acceptable. Only curved artery forceps should be used in these situations. If inserted with the curve facing into the wound a ligature may easily be slipped over the points and tied. Alternatively, the vessel may be dissected out and widely spaced ligatures placed around it before division. Any ligature too close to the point of division may slip at a later time and lead to unexpected bleeding (Fig. 4.16). For small vessels a twist of the artery forcep is often enough to seal the vessel. If a tie is not deemed adequate the vessel may be formally oversewn or transfixed with a heavy suture (Fig. 4.17).

Use of local anaesthetics with adrenaline, adrenaline solutions alone or POR 8 will also reduce bleeding in these layers. In certain types of distal limb surgery an arterial tourniquet may be used. This will render the distal part of the limb totally ischaemic and prevent blood obscuring the operative field in any procedure where loss of vision may be disastrous. Unfortunately, the potential side effect of this apparatus is that

Artery forceps are placed on the vessel with the curved tips pointing towards each other. The vessel is then divided.

(a)

(b)

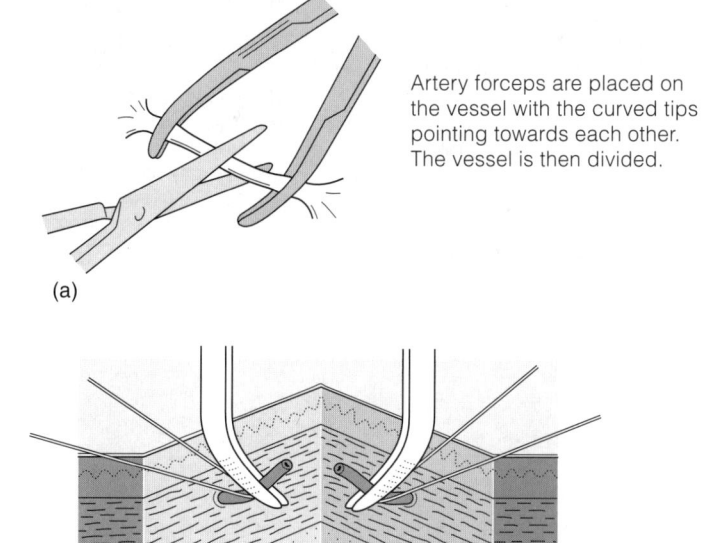

Threads are then placed around the vessel ends, behind the forceps, and the vessel ligated.

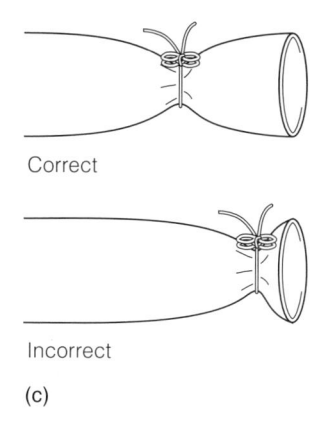

Correct

Incorrect

When ligating a vessel an adequate cuff of tissue must be left past the tie. An inadequate amount may allow the tie to slip off and bleeding to occur into the wound.

(c)

Fig. 4.16 *Vessel ligation*

Basic Surgical Skills

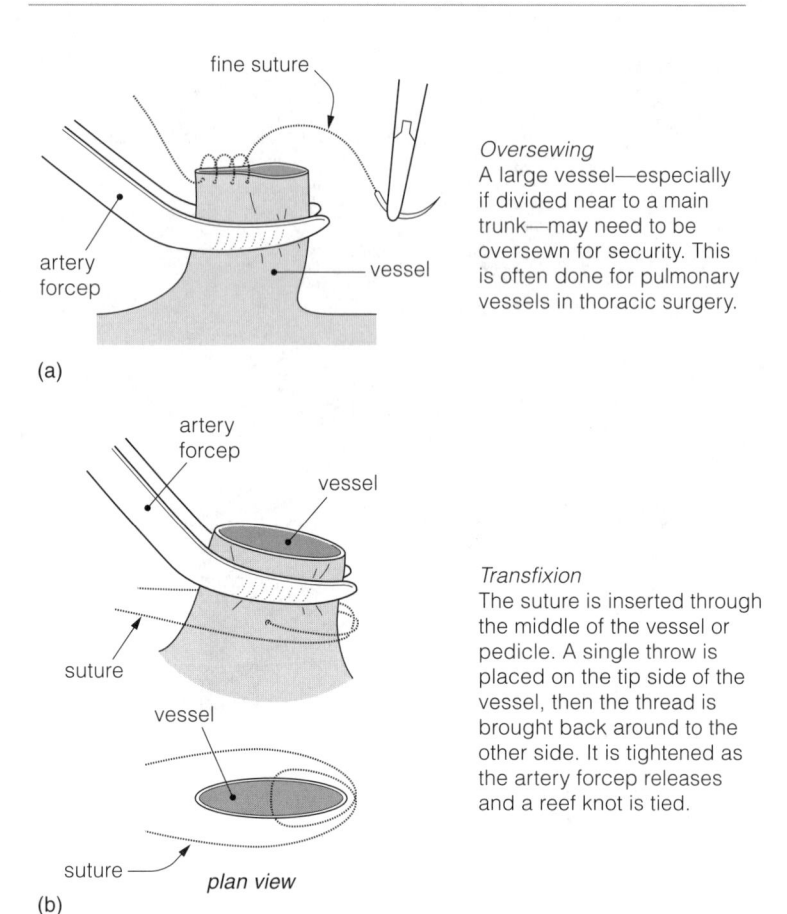

Oversewing
A large vessel—especially if divided near to a main trunk—may need to be oversewn for security. This is often done for pulmonary vessels in thoracic surgery.

Transfixion
The suture is inserted through the middle of the vessel or pedicle. A single throw is placed on the tip side of the vessel, then the thread is brought back around to the other side. It is tightened as the artery forcep releases and a reef knot is tied.

Fig. 4.17 *Oversewing and transfixion of vessels*

bleeding during the operation will be obscured. The subsequent lack of adequate intraoperative haemostasis may lead to postoperative bleeding, haematoma and a potential for infection.

When operating on, or adjacent to, major vessels these should be dissected and controlled with a rubber sling or vascular clamps. This will provide the maximum safety if damage occurs. A sling can be lifted and therefore tightened to occlude flow and a loosely positioned clamp may be easily closed (Fig. 4.18).

If control is not obtained and a major vessel is disrupted the best way to gain immediate control is to apply direct pressure. This is usually done with a pack and a hand but special instruments have

Basic Surgical Skills

(a)

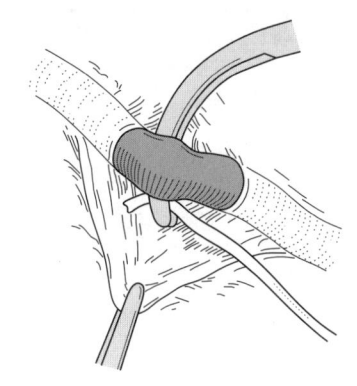

Inserting a silicon vascular sling: the right-angle forcep is used to dissect a tunnel behind the vessel and draw the sling through.

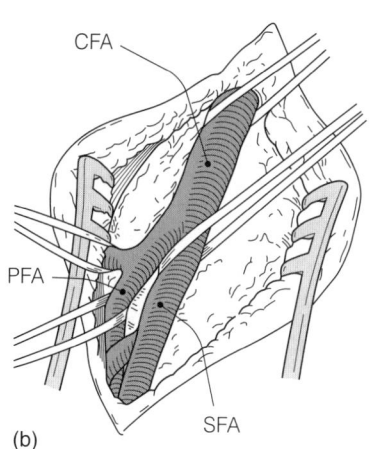

(b)

The right femoral artery complex with slings around the:
- common femoral artery (CFA)
- superficial femoral artery (SFA)
- branches of the profunda femoris artery (PFA)

The slings are inserted before applying the non-crushing vascular clamps.

Fig. 4.18 *Vessel slings*

been designed to occlude the aorta in these situations. If the bleeding is arterial, proximal pressure on the vessel is just as effective. Once controlled the damage can be repaired in most instances. Occasionally, however, the vessel must be tied off or, if not visible, the whole area from where the bleeding originates may have to be oversewn. While apparently drastic it is very unusual for an adequate collateral supply not to develop for the area that has lost its major vessel (Table 4.2).

Continued bleeding from a site where no individual vessels are found, or where the bleeders are too small and numerous to deal with (capillary oozing or venous bleeding), is exceptionally difficult to control quickly. Initial pressure with a pack, combined with progressive diathermy as the pack is slowly removed, will often alleviate this

> **Table 4.2 Methods of mechanical haemostasis**
>
> - Initial pressure with a pack
> - Progressive diathermy as the pack is removed
> - Application of haemostatic substances (topical thrombin, gel-foam, haemostatic gauze)
> - Ligation, transfixion or oversewing of bleeding vessels or areas
> - Packing and pressure left *in situ* for a period of time (tamponade)

situation. In more stubborn situations the application of haemostatic substances such as topical thrombin, gel-foam or haemostatic gauze may often help. If a large vessel or area of bleeding is observed it may be ligated, transfixed or oversewn. Sometimes a combination of packing and pressure is required to prevent massive bleeding, and on rare occasions these packs may be left in situ for several days before removal. This provides a tamponading effect and the packs can be removed at 48+ hours during a second-look laparotomy.

Postoperative measures

Although not strictly prevention, the monitoring of coagulation profile and blood components may be useful postoperatively. Appropriate measures can then be taken to replace blood being lost, correct coagulopathies and anticipate the need for reoperation if bleeding is excessive.

Basic dissection techniques

Dissection is the division of tissues required to approach, identify and expose an underlying structure or lesion. This process is required to facilitate the identification, display, examination, manipulation or excision of the particular structure/lesion.

Dissection may be undertaken in a *blunt* or *sharp* fashion. Blunt dissection involves pushing away, splitting, stripping, squeezing or other methods that separate the tissues without actively cutting them. Sharp dissection makes use of scalpels, scissors or diathermy to actively divide tissues in a very precise manner.

The process of dissection must be carried out with the maximum care for all involved structures. Good dissection requires a combination of abilities. An intimate knowledge of relevant anatomy is vital, along with an understanding of the spatial relationship between structures. The structure of connective tissues must also be appreciated so that correct

Basic Surgical Skills

planes and lines of dissection can be identified and entered. Experience with surgical dissecting techniques is essential, as this will ensure that appropriate decisions are made regarding the best method of dissection. Tissue trauma must be minimised by the gentle handling of both tissues and structures and, finally, tension (distraction of tissue) must be used appropriately to define the planes and expose the best lines of dissection.

Genuine skill in the area of dissection, then, is generally regarded as one of the hallmarks of general surgical competence (Table 4.3).

Table 4.3 Essential elements for successful dissection
- An intimate knowledge of gross and three-dimensional anatomy
- A knowledge of connective tissue structure
- An understanding of tissue planes
- Experience with various methods of dissection
- Minimisation of tissue trauma by gentle tissue handling
- The ability to use tension (distraction of tissue) in the display of tissues and planes

Blunt dissection

The simplest form of dissection is to follow the tissue plane that has been entered by pushing apart the tissues with fingers, gauze (pack, Raytec or peanut) or blunt instruments. This form of dissection does not involve the division of tissues, merely their separation. An important point in the performance of blunt (and sharp) dissection is the use of tension. By applying a 'distracting' (pulling apart) force to tissues they part with less direct force at the point of dissection. Tension will also help display the best line of dissection and simplify the decision of which method of dissection to use.

With fingers

Tissues may be 'torn' apart at their weakest point (usually a plane or line of cleavage) by applying a firm distracting force, from a distance and at an angle to the line of planned division. Unfortunately, this is an *inexact and often uncontrollable method* and may result in damage to adjacent structures. It is best avoided if possible.

The same process, with much less force, is the best way to provide tension for other methods of dissection. With tissue displayed in this way (Fig. 4.19a) the peeling away of layers by the insinuation of a finger or gauze peanut (pledget) on an instrument may be undertaken. The same effect can be achieved by the use of a hand-held pack or swab, or with a blunt instrument such as the reverse end of a scalpel handle.

A variant of this technique is the use of a hand- or instrument-held gauze swab to wipe away loose tissue layers from a structure that is itself being kept under tension. This is particularly effective in the dissection of layers of the spermatic cord during inguinal hernia repair (Fig. 4.19b).

Blunt dissection can also be used to divide tissues without damaging vital structures contained within them. Once again fingers can be used for the techniques of pinching and finger fracture. *Pinching* involves the squeezing of tissues between the thumb and forefinger to separate

(a) Push method

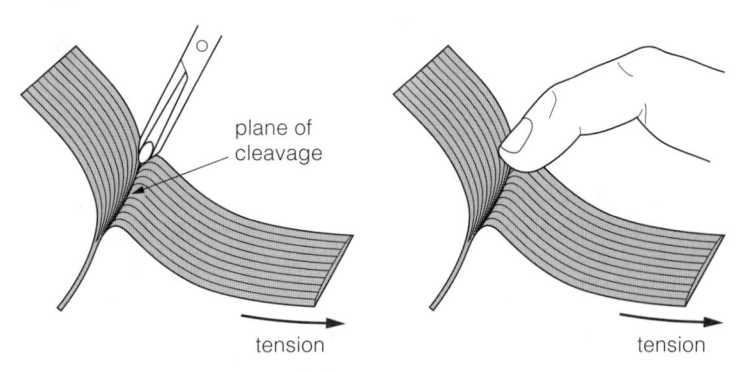

Tissue planes may be dissected by putting one element on stretch (tension) and then pushing a blunt instrument (finger or peanut swab) into the plane.

(b) Wipe method

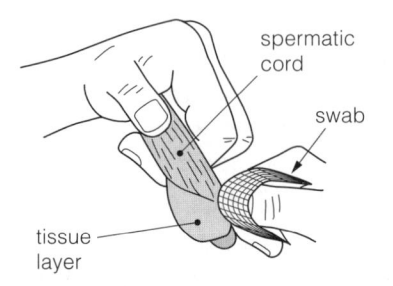

A gauze swab held between the thumb and forefinger of the right hand is used to 'wipe' away layers of the spermatic cord during a hernia repair.

Fig. 4.19 *Blunt dissection*

them along natural cleavage planes or lines of least resistance. This may be done to separate adjacent adherent tissues or to break through tissues such as the mesentery, or the oedematous fat in Calot's triangle during open cholecystectomy for acute cholecystitis.

A variant of this technique, called *finger fracture*, is used to dissect through friable vascular organs such as the liver. It has the advantage that homogeneous cellular material is broken down without disrupting blood vessels or bile ducts. These can then be separately clamped, divided and ligated.

With instruments

Blunt division of tissues with instruments relates mainly to dissection through a tissue *in the line of its fibres*. This process is usually referred to as *splitting tissue*. Muscle, aponeuroses and the connective tissue surrounding 'longitudinal' structures (nerves, vessels, bones and tendons) are all amenable to division by this method.

Two main variations exist within the technique of splitting. In the first, a pair of scissors is held in the semi-open position. One blade is inserted through the tissue to be divided. The scissors are then pushed along the line of the tissue, separating adjacent fibres. The open scissors blades will passively divide any fibres at right angles to this plane. This method is particularly used for aponeuroses and connective tissues as described above.

The second variation of splitting is when the scissors (or any opening instrument of scissor type) is inserted between the fibres of a structure and then opened to spread these apart. This manoeuvre may be performed in, or across, the line of the fibres. Once commenced it may be enlarged further by the use of retractors or fingers to spread widely the structure being divided. The opening of the abdomen for appendicectomy via a Lanz (oblique RIF) incision employs both forms of this splitting technique (Fig. 4.20a, b).

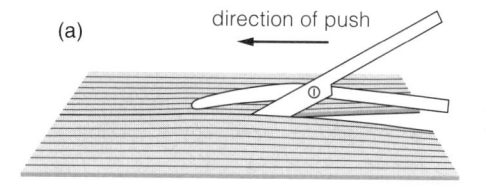

(a) direction of push

Splitting an aponeurosis in the line of the fibres with a partly open pair of scissors pushed along to split the fibres.

Fig. 4.20 *Splitting tissue with scissors*

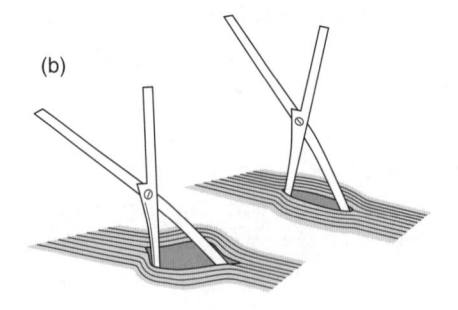

(b)

Muscle being split by scissors inserted between the fibres and opened *across* (left) and *in* (right) the line of the fibres.

Fig. 4.20 *Splitting tissue with scissors (cont.)*

Sharp dissection

Sharp dissection is the process of using a bladed cutting instrument to divide tissues in order to access deeper tissue planes or structures. The most common instruments used are scalpels, scissors (dissecting patterns) and the diathermy. All these instruments will divide along planes and through tissues with reasonable ease. Problems with cutting usually only occur when inappropriately small instruments are used for bulky tissues or the instrument is actually blunt. It must also be remembered that most scissors are designed for use in either the left or right hand, making dissection virtually impossible with the other hand.

The scalpel, which is discussed in previous sections, comprises a handle and a (usually) detachable razor-sharp blade. Its use as a first-line dissecting tool is not common but when held like a pen the scalpel is a very precise instrument. It will only incise tissues cleanly, however, if it can overcome the frictional drag of those tissues. If this is not achieved the tissues will pucker, drag and cut unevenly. The easiest way to overcome a problem with friction and drag is to provide stabilising tension either in the line of the incision or at 90° to it.

The main advantage of the scalpel is the minimal damage it causes to surrounding tissue. The cut it produces is clean and the depth to which it penetrates can be varied with pressure of the forearm. These benefits are often outweighed, however, by the potential it has for damaging deep structures in the line of incision. With this in mind the scalpel should be used sparingly and only in situations of extreme control or where no vital underlying structures exist.

Scissors are an excellent tool as they can be used for both sharp and blunt dissection, can dissect in planes and through structures and cause minimal adjacent tissue damage. The blades must be kept in contact while cutting or they will grab and crush the tissue to be incised. As the deep blade is often hidden from view all tissues should be thoroughly assessed for other structures (nerves, vessels, ducts etc) prior to performing the cut.

A monopolar diathermy, in the form of a single-bladed instrument or forcep, is merely an electrode with which to apply an oscillating current to the dissection plane. The current exits through a broad grounding plate on the patient's thigh, buttock or back. A continuous alternating current (Cut setting) causes high temperatures and tissue vaporisation that cuts tissue with little coagulating effect. Pulsed alternating current (Coagulation setting) desiccates the tissues and coagulates vessels. Each may be used alone or the two blended to provide features of both. Beware of monopolar diathermy in patients with pacemakers and with alcoholic preparation solutions due to the fire risk. Once again this method can be used to dissect along or through planes and tissues.

In view of both the cutting and heat-producing potential of diathermy it is advisable to insert an instrument, or even a finger, below the layers to be incised. This will protect deep structures from direct division and from the effects of the local heat generated. Such a technique is particularly useful when cutting rectus abdominus in a Kocher's incision (place an open packing forcep below it) or when incising linea alba after the initial scalpel incision (fingers are excellent here).

Basic assisting techniques

Surgical assisting is itself an art and should not be regarded as a boring prelude to learning how to operate. It is as physically and mentally challenging as performing the operation itself. The best assistant is usually one who knows the operation intimately and who can predict the next step that will be taken. Anticipation and preparation will ensure a smooth-flowing sequence of steps and this is the assistant's ultimate goal.

Assisting will also allow the assistant to learn a variety of technical nuances, when expected steps are achieved differently from usual, or replaced by a different step. The philosophy of surgical assisting comes down to one phrase: 'A good assistant makes the surgeon perform a good operation.' The assistant has two major duties—*exposure of the operative field* and the *performance of surgical tasks*.

Exposure relates to both the view and the physical access that the assistant creates for the surgeon. Retraction of tissues is the mainstay of this process and must provide both an adequate view of the operative site and access for hands and instruments. This process must be combined with appropriate light alterations, dabbing away of blood, suction, provision of traction for dissecting and holding instruments and sutures. However, the assistant must not relinquish exposure to perform these other manoeuvres. If available, the scrub-nurse may also be able to hold retractors or perform some of these tasks. Unfortunately, perfect exposure for the surgeon may lead to no line of vision for the assistant. While suboptimal, this is sometimes essential for the success of the operation.

The surgical assistant must also be able to carry out many surgical tasks. These include tying sutures, applying or removing instruments, cutting, stabilising, providing counter-traction for dissection, closing wounds with sutures and following sutures—to name but a few. An assistant who works with one particular surgeon will frequently find all these things becoming an automatic part of the operative routine.

The assistant must concentrate as hard as the surgeon on the task at hand. Inattention and frivolity will often disturb the surgeon's routine and lead to a slow and staccato procedure. A good assistant will also, politely, point out any relevant surgical or anatomical features of a procedure that they feel the surgeon may have missed. It would be awful to watch an operation go horribly wrong when one short sentence from you may have prevented the irreversible manoeuvre. The surgeon should guide general discussion during the procedure and relevant questions are best asked only at rest, or at low-stress points of the operation. If asked an opinion on the situation at hand it should be presented concisely together with the reasoning behind it.

All this must be done while resisting any temptation to try to help the surgeon by performing parts of the operation. Dissection, or the undertaking of any part of the procedure, without an express request from the surgeon is not only bad manners—it may be legally questionable and even detrimental to the patient.

Preoperative assistance

It is extremely useful for the surgeon if the assistant ensures the presence of correct x-rays, appropriate reports and test results. Assistance in moving and positioning the patient is also much appreciated by the surgeon and theatre staff. Insertion of in-dwelling urinary catheters is often delegated to the assistant and it is of great benefit to be familiar with this procedure in both males and females.

Prepping and draping are usually done by the surgeon, but the assistant or scrub-nurse may be required to do this on occasion. The exact pattern used is often a matter of the surgeon's personal preference and guidance is usually provided for assistants if they are required to do it. Once the patient is prepped and draped the operative field must be set up with diathermy, suction, light handles, self-retaining retractors and other instruments as directed.

Intraoperative assistance

Incision

Placing a pack on the skin and providing traction at 90° to the incision will assist the accuracy of this procedure. The pack may then be inserted into the edge of the wound and held with flexed fingers to compress bleeding points and provide further exposure and traction for incising. Resist the temptation to wipe with a pack—dabbing soaks up blood without disturbing clots on the end of vessels but wiping disrupts these clots and causes bleeding. The pack can be slowly peeled away as the surgeon commences haemostasis. If an abdominal incision is being made, fingers or an instrument may be required to lift the peritoneum or anterior abdominal wall as the incision is continued superiorly and inferiorly.

Retraction

Retraction may be provided with tissue-holding forceps or purpose-built retractors. The art of retracting is a combination of gently displacing the tissues without causing damage and minimising energy expenditure so that the retractor arm does not fatigue and exposure is not lost. Once placed, try to keep a retractor in that exact position as it will usually be providing the best exposure. If you feel the retractor is about to move, inform the surgeon; they may wish to stop what they are doing to prevent inadvertent damage and reposition the instrument. If a surgeon takes hold of the retractor, let the instrument go immediately—this action usually means that they wish to reposition the blade.

The assistant should move the retractor only if specifically told to do so, if a suggestion for better exposure is accepted or if it follows the pattern of dissection or suturing—for example, along the edge of a mastectomy wound. Any movement of the retractor must be delayed until the surgeon is not cutting or suturing. A loss of vision caused by movement of the retractor may result in accidental damage to a vital structure. Special precautions must also be taken with long retractors, especially those with a posteriorly angled lip. Any excessive pressure, or toe-in movements from lifting the handle, may cause damage to deep structures such as liver, spleen or mesentery (Fig. 4.21).

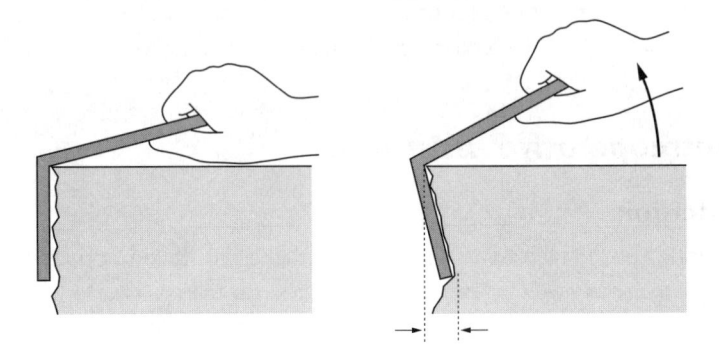

The effect of raising the hand with the bend of the retractor as a fulcrum is demonstrated. A significant increase in retraction is achieved with minimal increase in force. Care must be taken not to damage structures near the tip of the retractor.

Fig. 4.21 *Retraction*

Good retraction does not necessarily involve excessive force. Merely preventing the ingress of tissues by having the retractor in the correct position is often enough to give excellent exposure. If this is not adequate the judicious raising of a hand, with the bend of the retractor as the fulcrum, will often retract structures much further with less force. Care, as outlined in the previous paragraph, must be taken with this manoeuvre.

Table 4.4 summarises points to consider when retracting tissues.

Tension

Firm and gentle traction of tissues at 90° to the line of incision or dissection will often provide the surgeon with an obvious line or plane to follow. It will generally focus the greatest force on this line, thereby allowing those tissues to be divided most easily. The tension will also distract the tissues manually and assist with their physical separation. Application of tension may be achieved with retractors, hands, tissue

Table 4.4 Points to consider when retracting tissues

1. Gently displace the tissues without causing damage.
2. Minimise energy expenditure and reduce fatigue so exposure is not lost.
3. Retain exactly the position the surgeon has placed the retractor in.
4. If the surgeon takes hold of a retractor, let go—he wants to move it.
5. Only move the retractor if:
   - told to do so
   - your verbal suggestion to improve exposure has been approved
   - it follows the pattern of dissection, e.g. along the edge of a wound
   - the surgeon is not cutting—loss of vision may result in accidental damage to a vital structure.
6. Be careful with the toes of long retractors as excessive pressure caused by pulling or 'toe-in' movements may damage deep structures.
7. Good retraction does not necessarily involve excessive force. The judicious raising of a hand with the bend of the retractor as the fulcrum will often retract structures much further with less force (NB point 6).

forceps, hand-held forceps or a swab mounted on a sponge-holding forcep (*swab-on-a-stick*). Unfortunately, overly vigorous traction on tissues may result in uncontrolled tearing, bleeding and unnecessary damage. The gentlest possible force should be used and this can only be learnt through long experience.

Following

Holding the suture thread for the surgeon during suturing is termed *following*. It serves two main purposes. When a surgeon is creating an anastomosis, transfixing a vessel or vascular pedicle, oversewing bleeding sites or closing tissues there is often a need to maintain tension in the thread. This prevents suture slip and therefore laxity or gaps in the sutured tissue. It also keeps loose thread from encroaching on the tissue to be sutured as well as lifting and presenting these tissues for the next suture bite.

The correct technique for following a suture involves certain practical considerations. When taking the suture from a surgeon it should be pulled only at the same pressure and angle at which it was given. This will prevent inadvertent ischaemia by overtightening the stitch, it will keep the tissues best displayed, and remove you and the suture from the surgeon's line of view.

The suture should be held '60–40'—that is, 40% of the suture between the assistant's hand and the last stitch and 60% between the hand and the needle holder. This allows enough laxity for the surgeon to insert the next suture without excessive suture obscuring the view or tangling with the next bite. As the suture is pulled tight after each bite the assistant should allow the thread to run gently through the fingers. As it nears the end, following the thread all the way down to the tissue being sutured before release will keep the tension on the previous bite and allow this bite to sit in good position.

The thread should be observed carefully in order to prevent tangling in instruments or other fixed structures (known as 'locking-up'). Locking up the thread may cause breakage or damage to tissues as it is pulled tight.

Tying and suture skills

The assistant only rarely has to tie sutures but this is occasionally required in thyroid procedures or when the angle is unfavourable for the surgeon to tie. More commonly, the assistant will be required to steady and present an artery forcep for tying around. To do this well, the handles or arms of the instrument should be held in a comfortable position that presents the tips of the instrument for the thread to be slipped around. The instrument should not be pulled upwards as this may tear the vessel or tissue being tied, allowing it to retract and present further difficulties to control.

As the surgeon begins to tie, the forcep should be angled to allow the easiest access for tightening the knot. While doing this the assistant's hand and arm should be kept out of the surgeon's line of sight. When (and only when) asked, release the forceps slowly and gently and remove them from the surgeon's line of sight. If asked to *ease-and-squeeze*, gently release the forceps, leave them in position and reapply them once the first throw of the knot has been tightened. This manoeuvre allows control to be retained on the structure being tied and a second tie to be applied for further security if required.

When cutting sutures the scissors should be stabilised on the other hand, or another steady point, and the thread cut with the tips of the blades. This will ensure that no adjacent structures are cut and that the suture is trimmed to precise length. In general, a tag end of 3–6 mm should be left, depending on the size of the suture. Any longer than this and it may tangle with another stitch or present a foreign body for infection. Any shorter and the knot may unravel, leading to potentially disastrous consequences.

Haemostasis

The ingress of blood on the operative field is a great distraction to the surgeon. It obscures the view of the operative field and makes any manoeuvre hazardous until cleared away. There are several methods for removing pooling blood prior to adequate haemostasis being obtained.

A sucker may be used to remove blood from the operative field. The most common is the Yankauer sucker but other styles and sizes are available depending on the procedure. These are usually connected to high-pressure suction from the wall suction inlet, via a collecting bag system. It is a very rapid method of removal but has the disadvantage that it may dislodge a clot and actually worsen the bleeding problem.

As an alternative the *swab-on-a-stick,* a gauze swab wound around a sponge-holding forcep, is effective for small amounts of bleeding such as that on the bowel edge during an anastomosis. It is used to dab bleeding in these small areas and doubles as an effective retractor or as an instrument to put tension on tissues being dissected.

The placing of a pack into a bleeding wound will soak up free blood, tamponade bleeding while *in situ* and pull out any free clot when removed. The disadvantage of this is that the flow of operating must cease while in place. It is a very effective method, however, for cavity bleeding such as in the pelvis.

Wound closure

The process of wound closure involves most of the skills mentioned above including tissue retraction, following the suture, assistance with tying and blood removal. The one special skill is in the insertion of skin staples. There are many methods of insertion but one of the commonest requires both surgeon and assistant to pick up adjacent edges of the wound with toothed forceps. They both evert the edges and hold them together while the staple is inserted. This process is then repeated about one centimetre further on until the whole wound is closed. Alternatively, the surgeon may pick up both wound edges together with a heavy forcep in one hand and insert the staples with the other, in a manner similar to inserting Michel clips into a thyroid wound.

Postoperative assistance

Once the incision is closed the area is washed and dried, a dressing applied and drains secured with dressings and tape. The assistant should remain sterile and assist with these procedures. Assistance in moving the patient is, once again, greatly appreciated by all staff. The surgeon or assistant should take responsibility for all catheters and drains during this procedure. One or both should then follow the patient into recovery to ensure all is well. It is only when the patient reaches the PACU safely that the 'true', traditional assistant's job is at an end.

Further reading

Kyle J, Smith J & Johnston D, eds. *Pye's Surgical Handicraft*, 22nd edn, Butterworth–Heinemann, Oxford, 1992. Chap. 10, Assisting at Operations.

Kirk RM. *Basic Surgical Techniques*, 4th edn, Churchill Livingstone, Edinburgh, 1994. Many of the chapters deal, in greater depth, with the topics covered in this chapter.

Dudley DG. 'The Surgical Assistant', *Surgery, Gynecology and Obstetrics*, vol. 115, August 1962, p. 245.

Thompson RVS. *Primary Repair of Soft Tissue Injuries*, Melbourne University Press, Melbourne, 1969. Chap. 6, Lacerations without Skin Loss.

Thompson S. *Super Suturing*, Davis and Geck, Australia, 1991.

Zederfeldt H & Hunt T. *Wound Closure—Materials and Techniques*, Davis and Geck, USA, 1990.

Ethicon Sutures, *Wound Closure Manual*, Johnson & Johnson, USA.

The last three books are available through the appropriate company representatives that service your hospital or area.

Local anaesthetics and their uses

Introduction

Nerve cells (neurones) transmit electrical impulses. Motor nerves take impulses generated in the brain and conduct them to an effector (usually muscle) cell in order to perform a function. Sensory nerves conduct in the reverse direction, from a receptor in the periphery to the brain, allowing perception of a stimulus. The basis of local anaesthesia is to prevent perception of a noxious stimulus in the periphery (e.g. wound repair or excision of a lesion) by blocking impulse conduction along sensory nerves.

Nerve cell conduction relies on a process of local depolarisation and repolarisation across the cell membrane, which progresses from the point of stimulus origin to the next synapse. Cellular depolarisation is caused by a rapid movement of sodium ions *into* the cell from outside. Repolarisation of the cell is caused by potassium ions *exiting* the cell and a steady state is returned by special *membrane pumps* that return the translocated ions back to their original position inside or outside the cell (Fig. 5.1).

Local anaesthetics are a heterogeneous group of substances that prevent electrical conduction along neurones. As they are poorly

Local anaesthetics and their uses

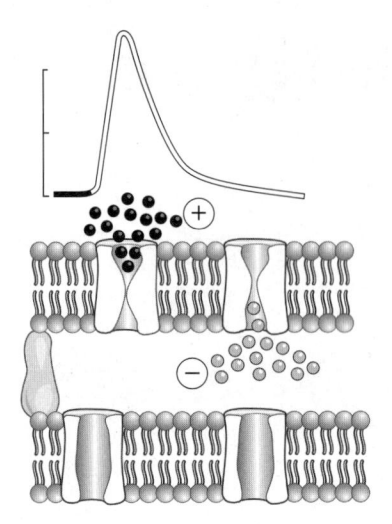

(a) Resting potential—positive outside the cell and negative inside.

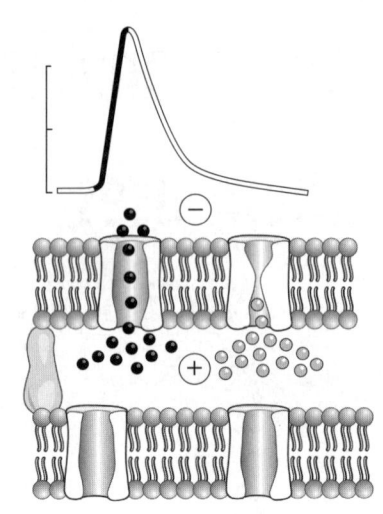

b) Threshold potential is reached, sodium channels open and positively charged (Na$^+$) ions flow into the cell depolarising the membrane.

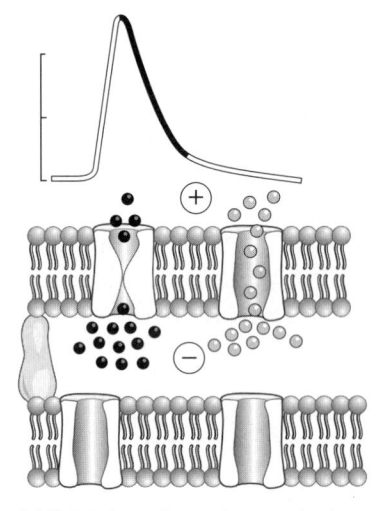

(c) Potassium channels open and positively charged ions (K$^+$) flow out of the cell to repolarise the membrane back to resting potential level.

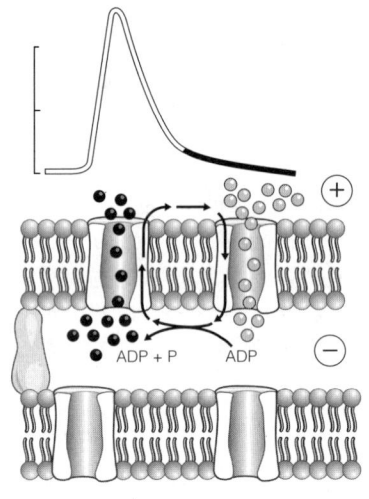

(d) An active transport mechanism transports sodium out of the cell and potassium back in. This restores the correct balance of ions inside and outside the cell while maintaining resting potential.

Fig. 5.1 *Nerve depolarisation and the mechanism of action of local anaesthetics*

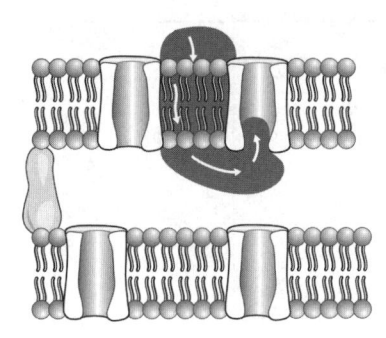

(e) Local anaesthetic enters the nerve cell via the cell membrane and blocks the ion channels from within the cell. This prevents conduction of impulses along the nerve. Anaesthesia occurs in the region supplied by the sensory axons of the blocked nerve.

Fig. 5.1 *Nerve depolarisation and the mechanism of action of local anaesthetics (cont.)*

water-soluble and bases, the active anaesthetic is in the form of a hydrochloric salt. They act by transiently 'blocking' sodium transport channels in the cell membrane. This prevents initial depolarisation of the cell at that point and is referred to as *membrane stabilisation*. The result is an inability of the neurone to reach threshold potential, at which it depolarises, within the region of local anaesthetic effect. As a consequence, the conduction of electrical impulses is interrupted and the neurone's function temporarily impaired or halted. Sensory neurones are more sensitive to this process than motor neurones. The overall aim of local anaesthesia, then, is to block local or regional sensory neurones with minimal effect on motor function.

There are many procedures, from caesarean section to craniotomy, that could be performed under local anaesthesia. Administration methods are also varied, ranging from the infiltration of tissues and nerves to local anaesthetic injections around the spinal nerve roots or spinal cord (see Table 5.1 and section below). In general, however, most practitioners will only ever use local anaesthetics for the repair of minor wounds or local excisions. Local infiltration to augment analgesia during or after general anaesthesia, in procedures such as hernia repair, appendicectomy and breast surgery, is also well recognised. The more advanced uses of local anaesthetic should remain solely within the province of specialist anaesthetists.

Table 5.1 Local anaesthetic uses

Method	Mechanism	Site of action and extent	Advantages / Disadvantages	Example
Topical administration	A lipid soluble cream, containing local anaesthetic, is applied to the skin. It is absorbed and blocks dermal neurones.	• Local tissues • Up to several millimetres deep	A – Simple and effective D – Shallow penetration	Local anaesthetic cream applied to the skin prior to an injection in children
Local infiltration	Local anaesthetic is flooded into the tissues and blocks all small nerves in the region.	• Minor sensory nerve branches and receptors • Full extent of the infiltration and subsequent diffusion	A – Simple and effective Adrenaline aids haemostasis and prolongs effect Hydro-dissection D – End-artery risk with adrenaline Obscured view Rapid offset with no adrenaline	Local injected around a skin cancer before excision
Nerve or plexus block	Local anaesthetic injection around a major nerve or nerve plexus diffuses around and into the nerve to block all fibres.	• Neurones of large nerves • The entire distribution of all nerves infiltrated. Does have motor effect as well	A – Very effective with long action and no other anaesthesia needed D – May fail and require GA Toxicity with accidental IV injection	Median and ulnar nerve blocks to anaesthetise the hand. Brachial plexus block in the axilla to anaesthetise the arm
Intravenous block (Bier's block)	Intravenous injection of local anaesthetic in an exsanguinated and arterially tourniqueted limb. Back flow through the veins into capillaries and ECF leads to tissue level anaesthesia.	• All nerve tissue within the limb • The entire limb below the tourniquet. Motor and sensory effect.	A – Rapid and effective Simple technique D – Potential toxicity as IV Exsanguination and ischaemia Special equipment required Occupies two doctors	Injection of local anaesthetic into the upper limb veins, after tourniquet and exsanguination, to anaesthetise for reduction of a Colle's fracture

Local anaesthetics and their uses

			A / D	
Centrineural block	Injection of local anaesthetic into the spinal column to anaesthetise at a central level. *Epidural*—outside the dura, bathes nerve roots in their dural sheath. *Spinal*—into the subarachnoid space to bathe the spinal cord and nerve rami inside their sheaths.	• Epidural—on the spinal nerve roots • Spinal—directly on the spinal cord and nerve rami • Multiple dermatome levels as the local anaesthetic diffuses along planes	A – Rapid and very effective Simple to administer Postoperative analgesia too D – Failure rate and patient discomfort Injury to spinal cord / nerve roots Dural puncture Bacterial inoculation/abcess Sympathetic blockade Respiratory effect/high spinal	Single administration of local into the subarachnoid space to anaesthetise the lower abdomen for inguinal hernia repair. Placement of an epidural catheter for augmenting anaesthesia during, and providing analgesia after, a major abdominal procedure
Cavity administration	A catheter is placed into a wound or cavity (e.g. pleura) for intermittent or continuous administration of local anaesthetic as an analgesic	• All local nerves in a wound and nerves, in the region of cavity administration, that the anaesthetic can diffuse to • As far as the anaesthetic diffuses or spreads in the cavity	A – Simple and can be effective D – Failure rate and patient discomfort Bacterial inoculation	Placement of a catheter into a subcostal (cholecystectomy) wound for postoperative analgesia

Local anaesthetics and dosages

Two distinct families of local anaesthetic exist—esters (of various substances) and amides. The latter are more commonly used in day-to-day practice. The main difference between the two lies in their metabolic degradation. Esters are hydrolysed in plasma by pseudo-cholinesterases and amides are metabolised by the liver. Both types act to block sodium channels in the cell membrane of neurones.

The most frequently used local anaesthetics in non-specialist anaesthetic practice are lignocaine (lidocaine in the US), bupivicaine and prilocaine. Each has specific properties that make it most appropriate in certain circumstances and all are available in a variety of concentrations, from 0.25% to 2%. There are also combinations of these with adrenaline in concentrations from 1/100 000 to 1/400 000. A newer local anaesthetic, ropivicaine, has recently been released and is now finding its place in clinical practice.

The safe dose of any local anaesthetic can be affected by many factors and so may vary considerably between individuals. It is usually expressed in terms of a 'milligram per kilogram body weight' dose. An exact volume available for administration can then be calculated by knowing the concentration of the anaesthetic solution. The main factor in deciding dosage regimes is the known toxicity profile of an individual drug. This usually has a fixed maximum value that should only be exceeded by experienced personnel.

Other dose-altering considerations include the site and method of administration, the co-administration of adrenaline or other vasoconstrictors and the speed of administration. These factors are dealt with more extensively in several of the recommended readings.

The required rapidity of onset and duration of action are factors that may affect the choice of drug. These parameters are also dependent on site of administration, pH of the tissues and the co-administration of vasoconstrictors. The faster amide anaesthetics, prilocaine and xylocaine, start working within minutes whereas esters, such as procaine and tetracaine, may take up to 18 minutes to commence their action. Similarly, duration varies greatly. Refer to Table 5.2.

Table 5.2 Common local anaesthetics and their properties

Drug	Dose (plain)	Dose (with adrenaline)	Onset (mins)	Duration (hrs)	Comments
Lignocaine	2–4 mg / kg	7–9 mg / kg	5–10 mins	1–2 hrs (plain) 2–3 hrs (adrenaline)	Commonly used as rapid onset and long enough for short procedures.
Bupivicaine	2.5 mg / kg	2.5 mg / kg	10–15 mins	3–4 hrs (plain) 3–5 hrs (adrenaline)	Slower onset with less motor blockade. More cardiotoxic than lignocaine and can precipitate arrhythmias.
Prilocaine	5 mg / kg (400 mg max / day)	5 mg / kg (400 mg max / day)	5–10 mins	1–2 hrs (plain) 2–3 hrs (adrenaline)	Rapid onset but much reduced toxicity. Can be used IV (Bier's block). Methaemoglobinaemia in high doses.
Ropivicaine	200 mg total	N/A	1–15 mins	2–6 hrs	No better or longer with adrenaline. Less cardiotoxic than bupivicaine.

Note: The doses in this table are approximate only and should not be used in place of the appropriate product information. Review the product information for each drug before prescribing.

Source: Compilation assisted by Astra Pharmaceuticals Product Information Literature

Local anaesthetic toxicity

Toxicity

As with all drugs, local anaesthetics have the potential to harm the patient through both known adverse actions (side effects) and unexpected reactions (allergies and idiosyncratic reactions). The non-allergic effects are usually dose-related and an overdose is usually (but not always) required for them to manifest. Overly rapid absorption and accidental intravenous administration of anaesthetic are the other major causes of adverse events.

There is often warning of impending toxicity as the effects are usually evident in the central nervous system first and follow a progressive and recognisable course. This should be understood and looked for by anyone administering local anaesthetics. Treatment can then be instituted before a significant adverse event occurs.

Non-allergic side effects occur mainly in excitable tissue because of the mechanism of these drugs. The neurological system is most commonly affected and it is only at the later stages and higher doses that cardiovascular effects become apparent. This is not always true of bupivicaine, which has a particular cardiac predilection. True allergic responses may occur but these are most commonly found in the ester group of anaesthetics. An allergy may also relate to preservatives or other chemicals within the vial. If there is any doubt, a properly supervised skin test should be performed (see Table 5.3).

Table 5.3 Reactions to local anaesthetic agents

Classification	Signs and symptoms
Neurological—early	Mouth and tongue numbness, tinnitus, anxiety, tremor and twitching, dizziness, confusion, drowsiness
Neurological—late	Fitting, coma, respiratory arrest, death
CVS	Hypotension, myocardial depression, cardiac arrest Cardiac arrhythmias with bupivicaine
Respiratory	Tachypnea or respiratory depression
Allergic	Nausea and vomiting, urticaria and anaphylaxis

Source: Compilation assisted by information from *Sabiston's Textbook of Surgery*, 15th edn, WB Saunders Co., Philadelphia 1997; and *Introduction to Regional Anaesthesia*, 2nd edn, Mediglobe SA, Fribourg 1995

Contraindications and precautions

There are some particular contraindications to local anaesthetic administration. These include known hypersensitivity to the anaesthetic, using prilocaine in anaemia or methaemoglobinaemia and administering bupivicaine for regional intravenous anaesthesia. The use of adrenaline-containing solutions in end-artery sites such as the fingers, toes and penis is also not recommended as it may lead to significant vasospasm and ischaemic necrosis of the part.

Other situations in which local anaesthesia must be administered with extreme caution include patients with shock, hypotension or hypoxia as these potentiate the toxic effects. Patients with pre-existing heart blocks or dysrhythmias are also more at risk from the cardiovascular side effects, especially those caused by bupivicaine. Liver disease, epilepsy and respiratory impairment should also result in greater caution.

Specific tips to prevent toxicity include:

- never exceed the recommended dose
- always pick the lowest toxicity alternative
- give it slowly and in small aliquots
- aspirate to ensure needles have not been accidentally inserted into a vessel.
- arrange skin patch testing if an allergy is suspected.

Patients undergoing local anaesthesia should be fasted and have intravenous access for emergencies, and full resuscitation facilities should be available. Finally, any patient undergoing an intravenous (Bier's) block should have two doctors in attendance—one to perform the procedure and one to administer and control the anaesthetic (see Table 5.4).

Management of toxicity

The earliest signs of toxicity will usually be central nervous in origin but any situation, up to a cardiac arrest, may be the first indicator of a problem (see Table 5.3). Prophylaxis is better than treatment but the administering doctor should be able to perform emergency life support and access assistance rapidly if required (see Table 5.4). Full CPR and the management of an arrest will not be dealt with here.

In situations where toxicity is suspected the first step is to administer oxygen by mask and ensure an adequate airway, and immediately postpone the procedure. Intubation and ventilation are rarely required for

Table 5.4 Safety considerations in local anaesthesia

Situation	Elements
Contraindications	• known hypersensitivity • prilocaine in anaemia or methaemoglobinaemia • bupivicaine for IV anaesthesia • adrenaline containing solutions in end-artery territory
Special caution	• shock, hypotension or hypoxia • pre-existing heart block or dysrhythmia • liver disease • respiratory impairment • epilepsy
Prevention of toxicity	• never exceed recommended dose • use lowest toxicity agent possible • use small aliquots • administer slowly, especially IV • aspirate needles to check if accidentally placed intravenous • arrange a skin hypersensitivity test if suspicious of a potential allergy
Precautions	• patient fasted if possible • intravenous access in all • full resuscitation facilities available • two doctors for any intravenous (Bier's) block • maintain verbal contact with the patient to be alerted early if CNS toxicity occurs • stop procedure if toxicity suspected • request urgent assistance if toxicity suspected
Toxicity management	• airway/breathing/circulation (ABC) • oxygen by mask • treat convulsions if prolonged • treat hypotension if detected • call arrest if urgent assistance required

Source: Compilation assisted by information from *Introduction to Regional Anaesthesia*, 2nd edn, Mediglobe SA 1995

this. If a convulsion occurs and persists for more than 20 seconds it should be controlled with an appropriate agent such as diazepam 5–10 mg by slow intravenous injection. Hypotension may require administration of a vasopressor. Experienced assistance, brought most promptly by calling a Code Blue (cardiac arrest or equivalent), should be sought if there is any evidence of potentially significant toxicity.

Administration methods

There are many techniques by which local anaesthetics can be used to achieve anaesthesia (see Table 5.1). The major method used by non-specialist practitioners will be local infiltration (see below) but the others are discussed for completeness. The descriptions are not extensive and further reading material can be found at the end of the chapter.

Topical anaesthesia

Gel or cream forms of local anaesthetics are used very effectively on both mucous membranes and the skin. Lignocaine spray may also be used on the pharynx and respiratory tree for endoscopic purposes, and lignocaine gel squirted into the urethra for painless catheterisation or instrumentation. Xylocaine and amethocaine creams are used for an hour under an Op-Site™ dressing to numb cutaneous sensation. This has particular application for minor split skin grafting and for both injections and intravenous cannulation in children.

The major advantages of this method are the simplicity and effectiveness. Unfortunately, the penetration of anaesthesia is shallow and so only applicable for cutaneous work.

Local infiltration anaesthesia

The basic tenet of this method is that local anaesthetic injected into the tissue to be operated upon affects local pain receptors and nerve fibres. This causes localised anaesthesia and permits painless surgery.

Major advantages of this method include its ease and effectiveness. The slowed absorption and dissipation of anaesthetic solutions containing adrenaline prolongs anaesthesia, postoperative analgesia and hence patient comfort. Haemostasis is augmented by the adrenaline and hydro-dissection, by the injected fluid volume, can simplify the surgery.

Unfortunately, the presence of adrenaline puts end-artery locations at risk of ischaemia. No adrenaline means more rapid offset of analgesia. Finally, the operative site, or lesion, may be obscured due to large volumes of injected fluid.

Nerve blockade

In this method of anaesthesia the local anaesthetic is injected, after anatomical localisation, directly onto a nerve or nerve plexus. This blocks the transmission of both sensory and motor impulses along the nerve. Blocks such as this are commonly used in limb, hand and foot anaesthesia. Digital and major nerve blocks, such as median, ulnar or posterior tibial are particularly effective in minor cutaneous surgery. Instructions for each are found in the local anaesthetic texts available in most emergency departments or from companies that produce the agents.

Brachial or other plexus blocks may be very effective but should only be performed by specialist anaesthetists trained in these techniques. Special short bevelled needles are used for plexus blocks to reduce complications.

Regional blocks are exceptionally effective and patients often require no other anaesthetic during their procedure. The long-acting agents that are used also provide excellent postoperative analgesia. Failure, however, effectively commits the patient to a general anaesthetic and all its risks. There is also a risk of damage to nerves and adjacent structures during insertion of the needle and of toxicity due to inadvertent intravenous anaesthetic administration, especially in brachial plexus blocks.

Intravenous (Bier's) block

Intravenous anaesthesia is uncommon and only really applicable to limb surgery. After exsanguination and application of two tourniquets the local anaesthetic prilocaine is injected into a distal limb vein. The volume used fills all veins below the tourniquet and flows back into the capillary bed and extracellular fluid. This bathes peripheral nerves in local anaesthetic and provides complete motor and sensory blockade. Once the procedure is complete, the tourniquets are sequentially deflated for slow controlled release of the prilocaine, which rapidly clears from the extracellular fluid of the limb.

This technique is particularly useful for fracture manipulation and distal limb surgery. It is rapid, simple and effective and may be performed in the emergency department. Toxicity is always a potential problem due to intravenous administration of the anaesthetic. Prolonged exsanguination and hence ischaemia may compromise the limb. Two doctors are mandatory for safety reasons and special equipment, including a dedicated arterial tourniquet, is required.

Centrineural blocks

The mechanism of a centrineural block is administration of local anaesthetic into the subarachnoid or subdural space of the spinal column. This fluid bathes both the spinal cord and nerve roots in the subarachnoid space (spinal anaesthesia) or the durally sheathed nerve roots in the extradural space (epidural anaesthesia). This provides widespread anaesthesia in the areas supplied by the neural levels affected.

The solutions of local anaesthetic required for these procedures are generally more dense (heavier) than cerebrospinal fluid (CSF) so spread is controlled by gravity and the curve of the spinal canal. Spinal anaesthetics are a 'single-shot' technique and find use in orthopaedics, urology and abdominal surgery. Epidural anaesthetics usually have a catheter inserted so that a mixture of anaesthetic and analgesic can be continually infused both intra- and post-operatively. The opiate component is used to block spinal pain receptors.

These two techniques are simple to perform, in experienced hands, and provide excellent operative anaesthesia and postoperative analgesia. Inherent in the techniques, however, is the risk of injury to adjacent structures such as nerve roots, the spinal cord and the dura. Dural puncture is planned in spinal anaesthesia but damage from the much larger epidural needle can cause significant CSF leakage and severe headache. Failure of the technique requires general anaesthesia and can be the cause of inadequate postoperative pain relief.

Hypotension from sympathetic nerve blockade is the most common complication of these procedures and merely requires adequate intravenous fluid administration to correct. Bacterial inoculation with subsequent abcess formation and paraplegia is devastating but incredibly rare. In a similar vein, respiratory compromise from a high spinal is also possible but uncommon.

Cavity infusion analgesia

While technically a method of postoperative analgesia this method of local anaesthetic administration should be mentioned. Catheters may be placed in a wound or cavity (e.g pleura) to allow bathing of the tissues in local anaesthetic. It is a simple technique but suffers from its lack of reliability. Fluid accumulation may provide a nidus for infection and introduction of bacteria through the catheter is a possible problem.

Local infiltration anaesthesia

This section describes some basic principles of administration for infiltration of local anaesthetics. Specific techniques of nerve blockade will not be discussed as these can be found in the appropriate reference texts and are basically an exercise in surface anatomy.

Timing

Injection of the local anaesthetic prior to scrubbing allows adequate time for it to act before the first incision is made. The longer this interval the more likely that adequate anaesthesia will be achieved. Bupivicaine, one of the slowest-onset anaesthetic agents, always requires this pause. The skin should be prepared with an alcohol swab or antiseptic solution on a gauze swab first.

Dilution

If a large area is to be infiltrated, dilute the anaesthetic in normal saline to increase the volume without risking toxicity. Bicarbonate solution is sometimes used as this will also reduce stinging and speed the onset, as both are worsened by solution and tissue acidity.

Needle

Unless otherwise indicated a #25 (orange) or #23 (blue) needle should be used for infiltration. These are fine enough to minimise discomfort but long enough to reach an adequate distance. The needle should never be pushed into the hub, as breakage will necessitate operative exploration for the remnant.

Aspiration

Before injecting any substance the needle must be aspirated to ensure that inadvertent intravenous placement has not occurred. This is a cause of toxicity and hence major potential morbidity and aspiration should be routine procedure for all practitioners who administer local anaesthetic.

Infiltration technique

Sufficient width of infiltration must be provided for adequate debridement and skin excision. Both dermis and underlying tissues should be infiltrated. Marking both the lesion and the extent of infiltration will facilitate the operation. If there is a clean open wound, injection through the virtually insensate subcutaneous fat will minimise patient discomfort (see Fig. 5.2).

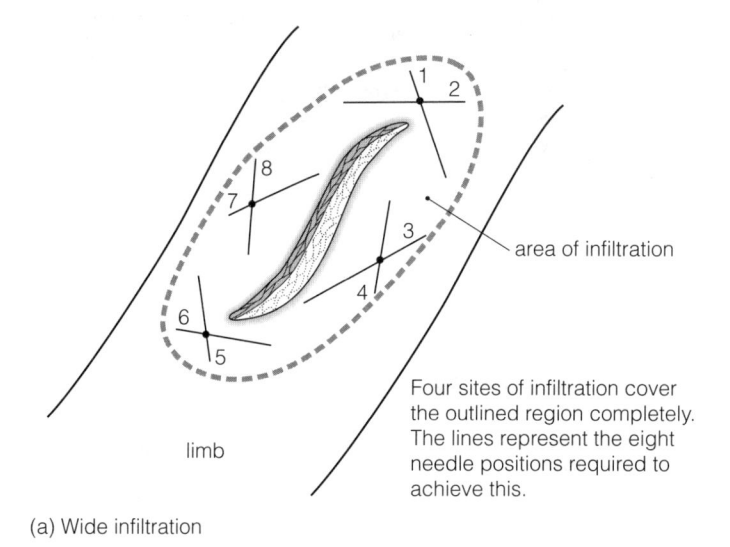

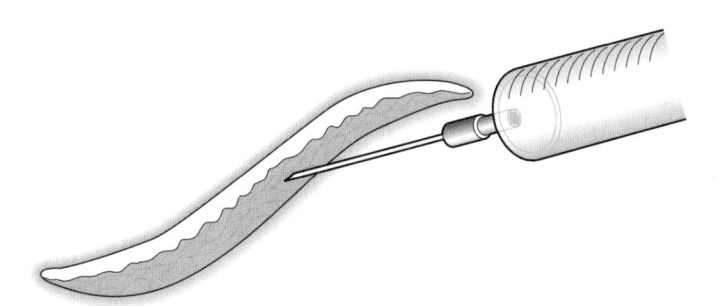

(a) Wide infiltration

area of infiltration

Four sites of infiltration cover the outlined region completely. The lines represent the eight needle positions required to achieve this.

limb

(b) Infiltration directly into subcutaneous fat results in less pain. This can only be done if there is minimal contamination.

Fig. 5.2 *Techniques of local anaesthetic infiltration*

Pressure

Firm pressure on the site of infiltration will stop bleeding and also help diffuse anaesthetic further through the local tissues. This reduces the difficult problem of lesions obscured by local anaesthetic blebs and increases the width of infiltration by diffusion.

Further reading

Cousins MJ & Bridenbough PO. *Neural Blockade*, 2nd edn, Lippincott, Philadelphia, 1987.

Scott D Bruce. *Introduction to Regional Anaesthesia*, 2nd edn, Mediglobe SA., Switzerland, 1995 (available through Astra Pharmaceuticals).

Wildsmith JAW & Armitage EN (eds). *Principles and Practice of Regional Anaesthesia*, Churchill Livingstone, Edinburgh, 1987.

Sterile technique

Introduction

One of the greatest advances in surgical science came with the introduction, by Lister, of an antiseptic environment for surgery. Influenced greatly by the germ theory of infection and work by Pasteur and others, Lister found that the use of carbolic acid spray in the theatre and on wounds significantly reduced the rate of infective complications. Unfortunately, carbolic had its own problems and even Lister himself admitted that the development of sterile technique was an improvement on, if only a logical extension of, his work.

The practical aspects of modern sterile technique have evolved significantly since Lister's time. Evidence has demonstrated that the measures employed prevent patient-borne infections as the consequence of an invasive procedure. An inevitable consequence of these measures is the reduction in *reverse contamination* and prevention of infection in clinical staff, by the patient.

Four main principles are embodied in the practice of sterile technique. These are adhered to most strictly in the operating theatre but also have application in procedures performed outside this environment. The first principle is *reduction of environmental contamination*. Easy within the theatre suite, this becomes progressively more difficult in the procedure rooms, wards and surgeries where sterile technique is also practised. In certain procedures, such as joint replacement and other prosthetic surgery, it is a vital point of practice, whereas in other situations it becomes less important.

The second principle, *disinfection of the procedural site*, is a virtually universal practice. Some evidence exists regarding special situations, such as urinary catheterisation, which suggests that disinfection is not as important as once thought. Nonetheless, this element of sterile technique does not compromise the patient and should be observed in all procedural situations to some degree.

The third principle, *isolation of the procedural site*, is maintained by the provision of barriers between the patient and both the proceduralist and the environment. These barriers prevent direct contamination of the patient from outside and contamination of the outside by the patient.

Sterilisation of procedural tools is the fourth principle. It is rare for this to be compromised but in certain situations, such as urinary catheterisation, its importance is less clear. Cleanliness, rather than sterility, is perhaps adequate for some procedures.

The main body of this chapter deals with the four principles of sterile technique in relation to operative surgery. While exceptions may exist in other procedural work, these four principles must be attended to in *all* operative situations. Failure to do so may compromise the patient, the proceduralist or other involved personnel and is unacceptable in modern surgical practice. A breach of these elements may even constitute malpractice and negligence on behalf of the proceduralist or hospital.

Table 6.1 The four basic elements of sterile technique

1. Reduction in contamination of the ambient environment
2. Disinfection of the procedural site
3. Isolation of the procedural site
   a) Provision of barriers between the proceduralist and the patient
   b) Provision of barriers between the patient and the environment
4. Sterilisation of procedural equipment

The principles and practice of sterile technique

This section looks at the four principles individually and highlights the specific practices and situations required for each. While this is by no means the final word in sterile practices, the aim is to provide a practical guide for all junior theatre personnel.

Basic Surgical Skills

Reduction of environmental contamination

When involved in theatre activities it is essential that all members of staff actively pursue the maintenance of an appropriately clean or sterile environment.

Clean staff

To maintain the *clean* environment of theatre, external dirt and contamination are minimised. To this end staff are required to change into clean theatre clothing before entering the suite. Hair and beards must be fully covered to prevent hair and debris falling in theatre. To prevent walked-in contamination street shoes must be covered with overboots, or special theatre footwear used. Masks are required in most theatres when sterile instruments are open to prevent droplet contamination (Fig. 6.1).

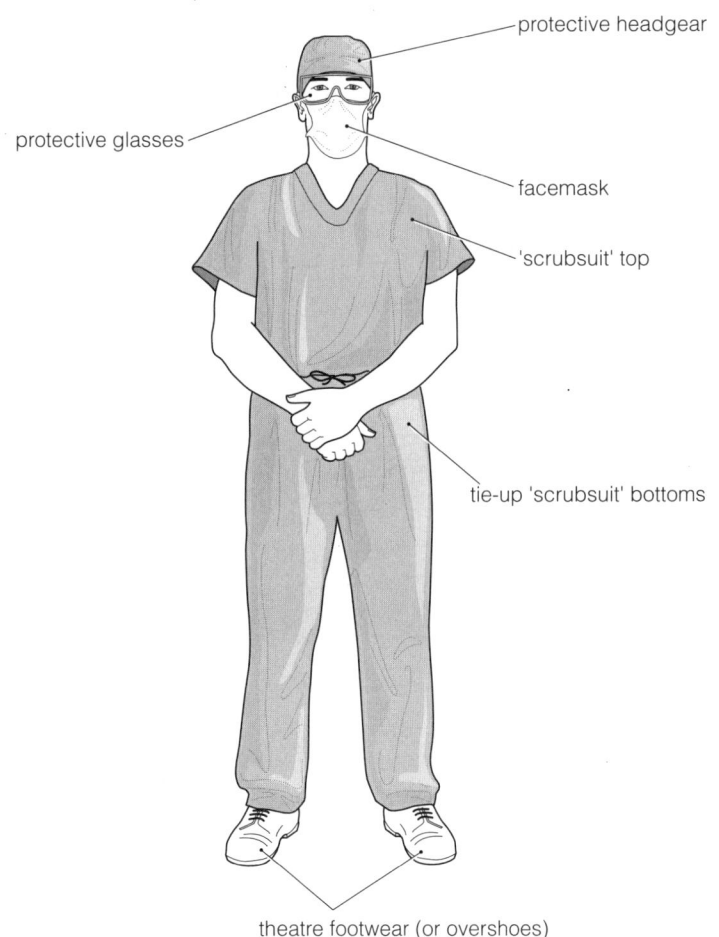

- protective headgear
- protective glasses
- facemask
- 'scrubsuit' top
- tie-up 'scrubsuit' bottoms
- theatre footwear (or overshoes)

Fig. 6.1 *Theatre staff member in clean apparel*

Clean air

Minimisation of draughts is thought to reduce the airborne contamination of wounds. Used particularly in orthopaedics, this concept has led to closed theatres for joint surgery, laminar airflow environments (filtered air directed down over the patient and away from the operative site) and minimisation of extra personnel and their physical movement within the theatre. Similar techniques should be used when possible for all theatres (Fig. 6.2).

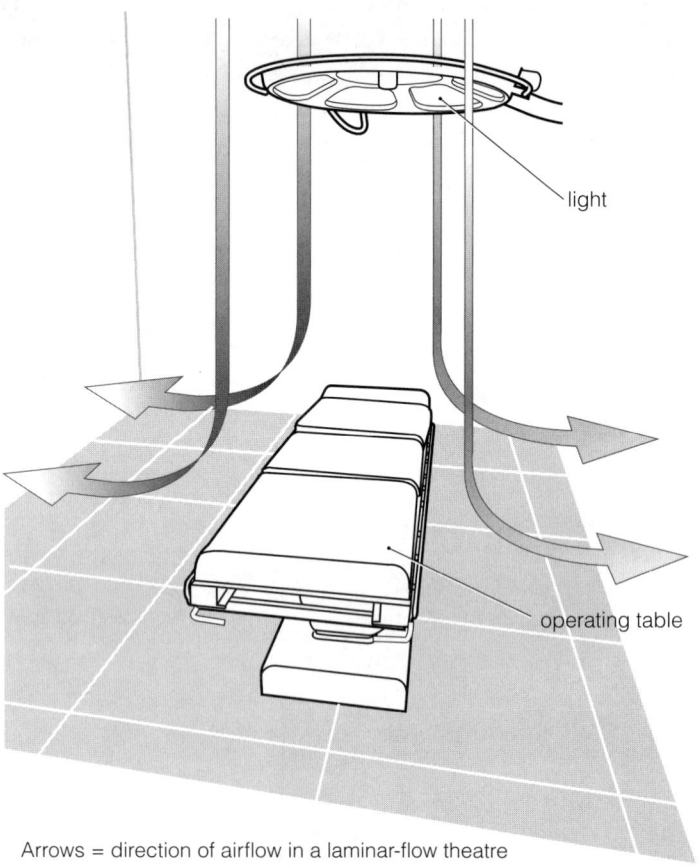

Arrows = direction of airflow in a laminar-flow theatre
- filtered air is blown down from above the table
- pushes particles away from patient
- air is extracted at the sides of the theatre

Fig. 6.2 *Laminar airflow as a technique for reducing infection*

Clean equipment

In general it is best policy not to touch any equipment in theatre unless you are required to. All staff should remain at least one metre from anything covered with sterile drapes. These items include draped patients, instrument trays and sterile trolleys. Sterile drapes are usually green or light blue in colour. If in doubt ask for permission to touch an object or move into a specific spot. It is much better to feel silly or sheepish than to contaminate a sterile field and bring the wrath of the scrub-nurse and surgeon upon yourself, or even put the patient's life at risk, with a single ill-considered act.

Instances of breaching sterile technique include leaning or reaching over sterile instruments and fields while not gowned and gloved, touching sterile personnel and trolleys, dropping non-sterile items onto the operative field or sterile trays. These actions happen particularly with novices in the theatre suite, such as medical students and student nurses, as they often do not possess the 'natural' responses that are required to avoid inappropriate contact and maintain the sterile environment. Contact with a sterile field is probably the commonest cause of a break in sterile technique by inexperienced personnel (Fig. 6.3).

Clean hands

All theatre staff should wear gloves during patient handling and wash their hands frequently to prevent cross-transfer of bacteria. This applies particularly to all members of the scrub team. Although there is little evidence to prove improved patient outcomes it is still recommended that all wash their hands and forearms with antibacterial solutions such as povidone-iodine or chlorhexidine. This is to reduce the resident bacterial flora present on the hand and upper limb, prior to gloving. The first scrub of the day should be for five minutes and the rest for three. This should encompass all the hand and forearm to elbow. If allergic to the wash substances, low-irritant antiseptics (such as Triclosan) and normal soap are acceptable alternatives. A summary of the Australian Confederation of Operating Room Nurses (ACORN) guidelines for the sterile surgical scrub is found in Table 6.2.

Disinfection of the procedural site

This refers to the process of cleaning, depilating and decontaminating the site of operation. Theatre technicians or nursing staff usually carry out the first two tasks. If grossly contaminated by dirt or grease a traumatic wound may first be washed, in a clean rather than sterile manner, to remove macroscopic contamination prior to skin preparation.

Basic Surgical Skills

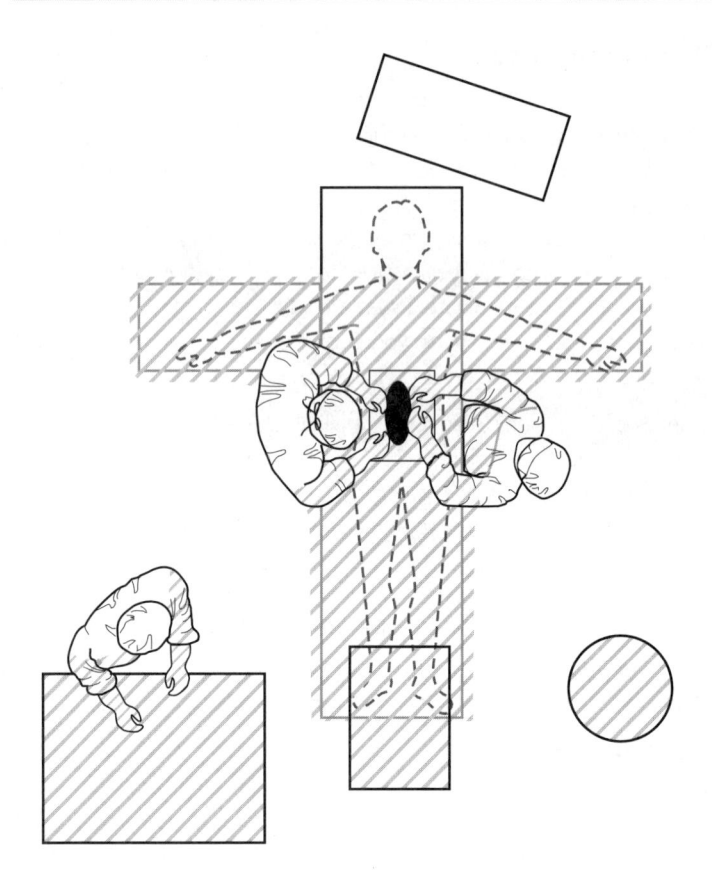

All green drapes, sterile trolleys, and the gloves, arms and thorax regions of sterile personnel are regarded as being sterile. Backs, shoulders and the fronts of gowns below the waist are *not* considered sterile.

Fig. 6.3 *Sterile areas on the operative field*

Once gowned and gloved, a member of the scrub team will paint the operative site with the antibacterial solution (prep). This should start at the site of incision and go outwards in circles of ever-increasing diameter. Swabs for prepping should be discarded when dry and new ones used. The old swab should not be re-dipped in the solution. A wider area than required should be prepped to allow for potential wound extension in unforeseen circumstances (Fig. 6.4).

Common preparation solutions include chlorhexidine (0.5%) in alcohol (70%), chlorhexidine (0.5%) and cetrimide (2%), 10% povidone-iodine solution, alcoholic iodine solution and aqueous chlorhexidine (0.5%).

Basic Surgical Skills

Table 6.2	Summary of ACORN guidelines for the surgical scrub	
Preparation	1.	Wear proper attire, cover hair, jewellery off, keep nails short, don mask and plastic apron.
	2.	Ensure presence of a sterile scrub sponge and antimicrobial wash solution.
The scrub	1.	Time scrub for 5 minutes (first for the day) or 3 minutes (all subsequent scrubs).
	2.	Wet arms to elbow under running water.
	3.	Wash with 2 ml of solution for 30 seconds with a circular motion; clean the nails, then rinse.
	4.	Wash again with 2 ml—between fingers up to elbow, and rinse.
	5.	Wash arms with 2 ml and rinse.
	6.	Wash hands with 2 ml and rinse.
	7.	Keep hands above elbows, turn off water and enter theatre with hands above elbows still.
Pre-gowning	1.	Dry hands and arms with a sterile towel—use a quarter for each hand and forearm.
	2.	Gown and glove as appropriate.

Source: Australian Confederation of Operating Room Nurses (ACORN) Standards Manual

All these have some amount of bactericidal action and all but the aqueous chlorhexidine overcome the skin's natural oils to 'stick' to the patient. Care must be exercised when using diathermy after alcoholic prep. The surgeon must ensure all the alcohol has evaporated or a spark may cause it to ignite. This is a well-documented complication that occurs *several times every year* in Australia (see Table 6.3).

Isolation of the procedural site

Draping the procedural site

Exclusion of the operative site with sterile towels or sheets is called *draping*. It is one of the barrier methods that protects the patient from environmental contamination. Sterile drapes may be made of cotton, paper or plastic and are usually held in place by a combination of gravity, friction and towel clips. Some of the disposable drapes have an adhesive layer that sticks them to the patient and occasionally a clear, sterile, adhesive plastic sheet is used to secure the cotton variety.

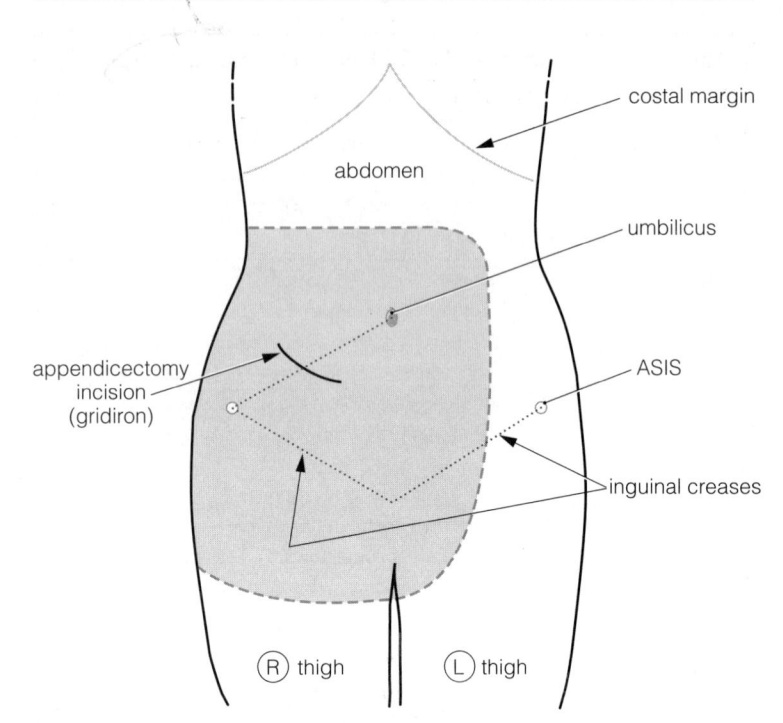

Despite the usually small nature of an appendicectomy incision a wider area has been prepared in case extension of the incision is required to deal with unexpected findings.

Fig. 6.4 *Example of wide skin preparation*

If waterproof drapes are not used a plastic sheet should be placed between the first layer of drapes and the patient to prevent fluid soaking through to the patient below. Any full-thickness saturation of drapes that contacts non-sterile material below causes a theoretical break in sterile technique.

In general the whole patient (except the head) is covered with drapes and two layers are the minimum standard at any point. A raised sterile curtain is usually placed between two poles to separate the anaesthetist and the surgeon. This protects both from contamination but is not practical in head and neck surgery. Only two draping techniques will be dealt with in this manual as many are intensely specific to each specialty and are often further personalised by individual surgeons; these are *square draping* and *shut-out draping*.

Table 6.3 Skin preparation solutions

Name	Contents	Uses	Precautions
Aqueous chlorhexidine	Chlorhexidine gluconate 0.05% w/v	General antiseptic and preoperative skin preparation	Should not contact eye, brain or middle ear Not for injection
Alcoholic chlorhexidine	Chlorhexidine gluconate 0.5% w/v in 70% w/w isopropyl alcohol BP	Hand rinse preoperatively or a preoperative skin preparation	Flammability; should not contact mucous membranes or brain, eye and middle ear Not for injection
Chlorhexidine and cetrimide	Chlorhexidine gluconate 0.015% w/v in cetrimide PhEur 0.15% w/v	General antiseptic and preoperative skin preparation May be mixed with aqueous chlorhexidine to reduce cetrimide concentration	As aqueous chlorhexidine
Povidone-iodine (aqueous)	Povidone-iodine 10% w/v (iodine and polyvinylpyrrolidone complex bound for slow release of iodine)	General preoperative skin preparation	Iodine hypersensitivity Long-term use in thyroid disease and lithium therapy Do not allow to pool on skin (burns) Not for injection
Alcoholic iodine	Iodine 0.5% in isopropyl alcohol 70%	General preoperative skin preparation	Flammability Iodine hypersensitivity Do not allow to pool on skin (burns) Not for injection

Source: Compilation assisted by information from data sheets contained in *Compendium of Data Sheets and Summaries of Product Characteristics*, Datapharm Publications Ltd, Great Britain 1998

Basic Surgical Skills

Square draping is the creation of a quadrilateral space containing the operative field within a combination of four or more drapes. This may be applied to the head, trunk and larger diameters of the limbs (Fig. 6.5). *Shut-out draping* is used to expose the distal part of a limb and involves a sterile base sheet, full preparation of the distal limb and application of a drape around the proximal limb to shut out the non-sterile segment (Fig. 6.6). A combination of the two methods may be required for the middle segment of a limb.

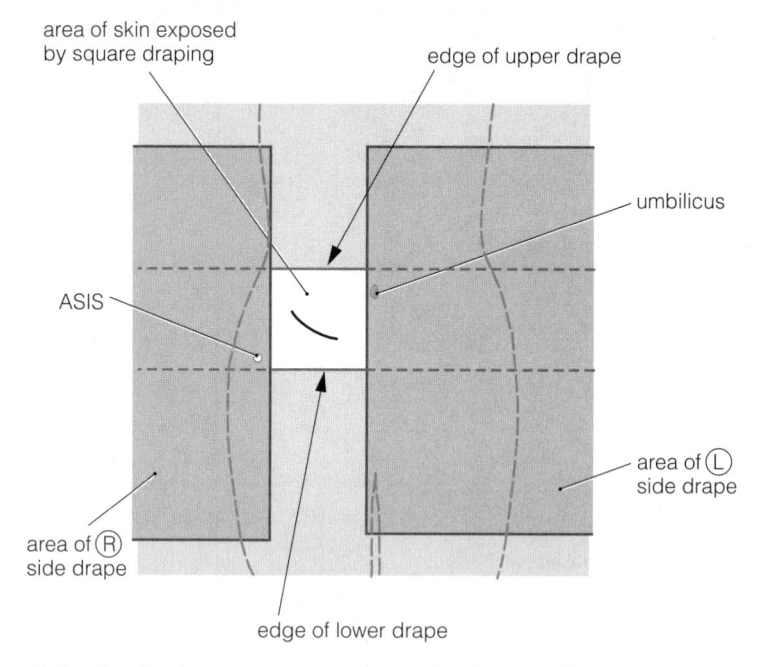

Notice that the drapes expose a wide area but there is still much more prepared skin available (see Fig. 6.4).

Fig. 6.5 *Square draping for an appendicectomy*

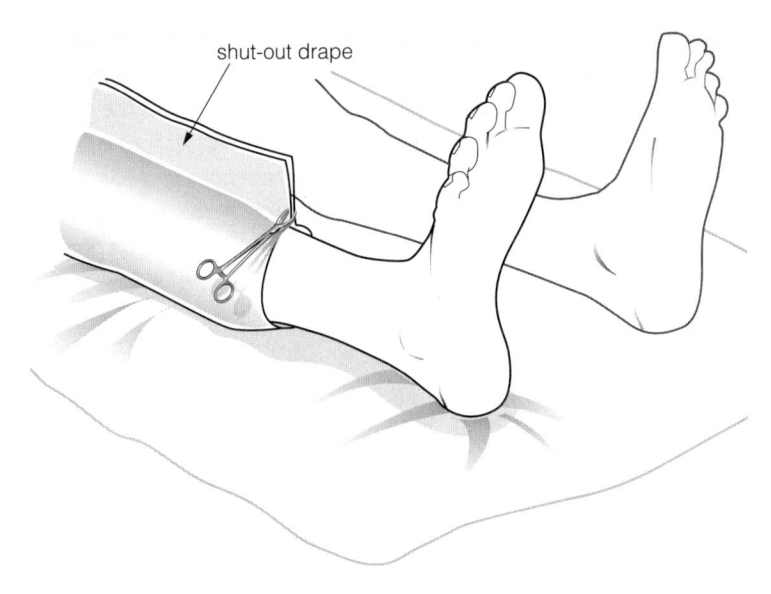

Fig. 6.6 *A shut-out drape positioned around the right calf*

Gowning and gloving

The use of barriers between the operative team and patient prevents transmission of infection in both directions. Gowns and gloves come in contact with the patient but masks, protective eyewear and 'space-suit helmets' do not. The entire surface of every gown and glove is fully sterilised prior to use, although the forearms, hands and chest region are the only parts of the theatre attire that are considered truly sterile. Contact, then, between other parts of the body and the operative field should be avoided as it creates a theoretical break in technique.

A summary of the ACORN guidelines for gowning and gloving is given in Table 6.4, with a visual guide in Figure 6.7.

Gloves are usually made of latex and come in sizes 5½ to 9. Different patterns and thicknesses of glove are available to suit individual needs and the type of surgery. Powderless gloves for abdominal surgery and powder-allergic personnel are available, as are neoprene gloves for latex-allergic staff and patients (see Table 6.5).

Basic Surgical Skills

Many personnel also choose to double-glove for all procedures (see Universal Precautions in Chap. 7). This practice does not prevent needlestick injuries in itself, and some would even argue that the potentially reduced sensitivity with double gloves in fact increases the risk. What double-gloving does do is provide a second, impervious protective layer over the skin. If a breach then occurs in the outer glove, and body fluid leaks through it, there is still protection for the skin. One study on double-gloving also showed a small but statistically insignificant increase in the

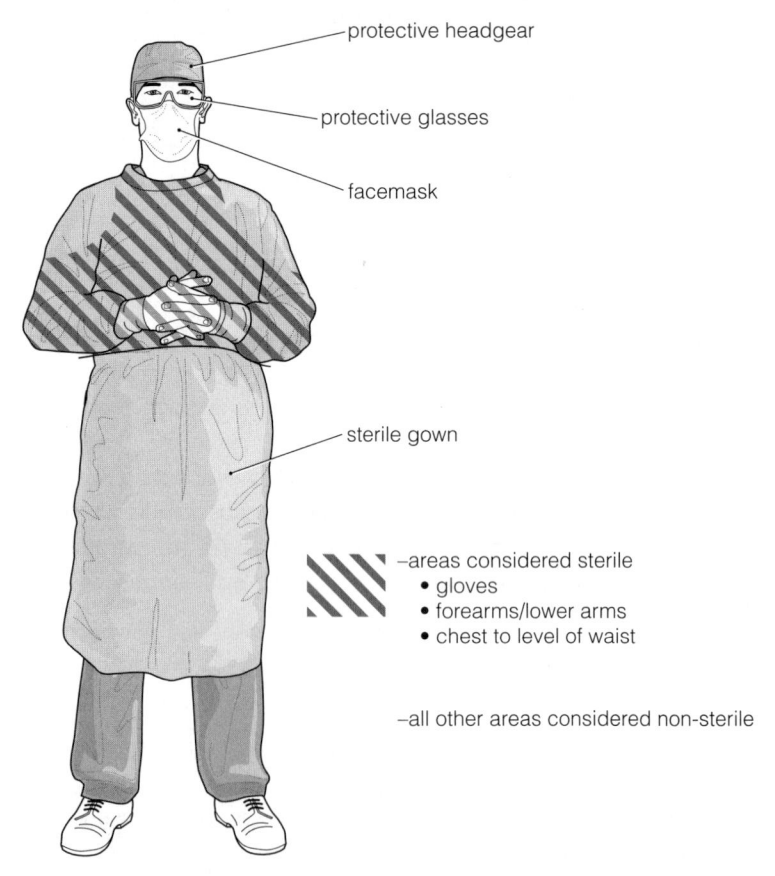

- protective headgear
- protective glasses
- facemask
- sterile gown

⧸⧸⧸ –areas considered sterile
- gloves
- forearms/lower arms
- chest to level of waist

–all other areas considered non-sterile

(a) Theatre staff member in sterile gown and gloves. Note the protective glasses, some form of which should always be worn.

Fig. 6.7 *Sterile gown and gloves*

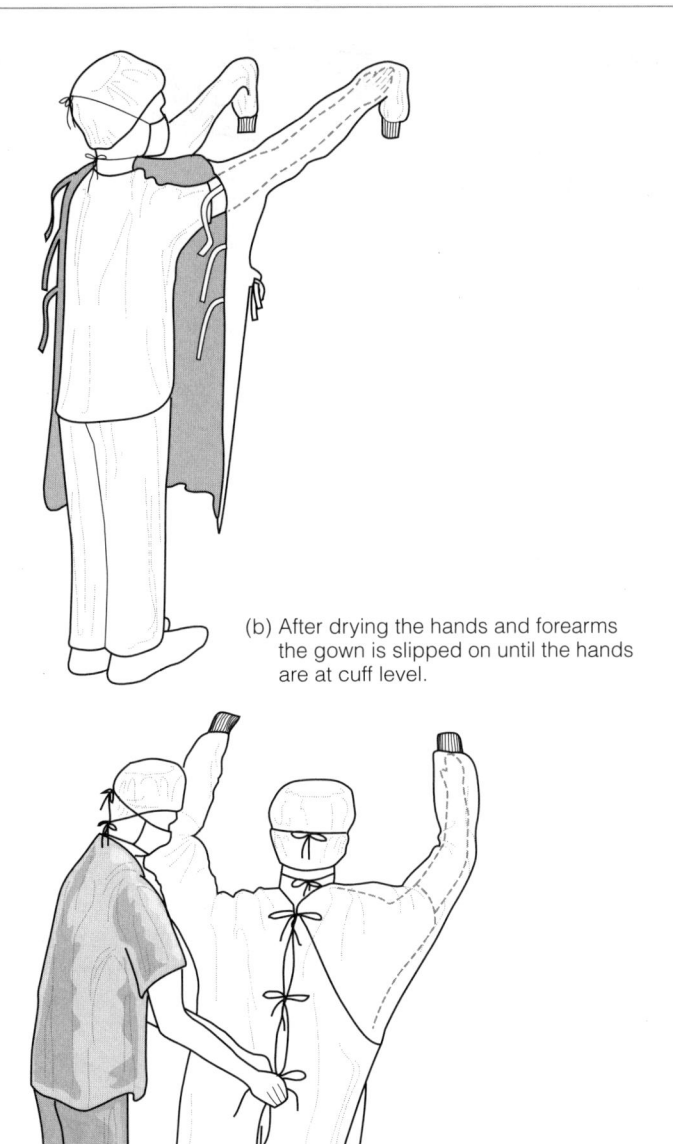

Basic Surgical Skills

(b) After drying the hands and forearms the gown is slipped on until the hands are at cuff level.

(c) With the hands still in the sleeves at cuff level the gown is tied.

Fig. 6.7 *Sterile gown and gloves (cont.)*

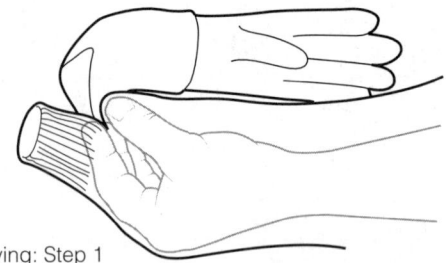

Basic Surgical Skills

(d) Gloving: Step 1

The glove is laid thumb-down on the forearm with the glove cuff gripped through the gown cuff.

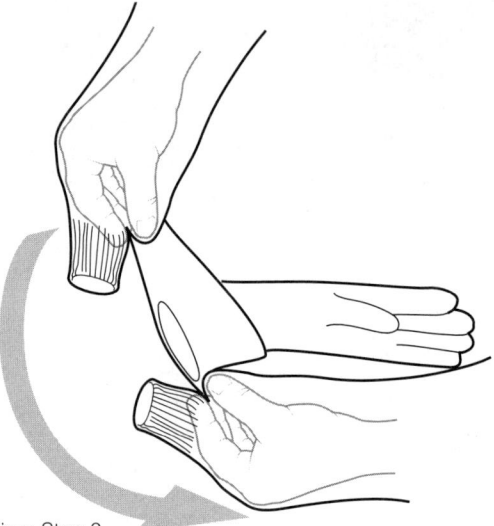

(e) Gloving: Step 2

The uppermost glove cuff is grasped through the cuff on the other arm. It is lifted over the open cuff end to effectively 'seal' the open cuff.

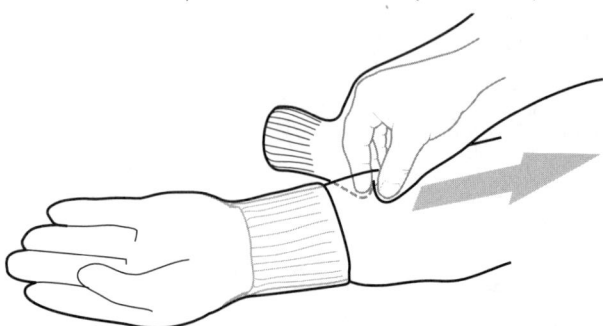

(f) Gloving: Step 3

Once the glove cuff is fully over the gown cuff, the other hand grips both and the hand slips into the glove against gentle counter-traction. Gloving is completed by performing the same steps on the other hand.

Fig. 6.7 *Sterile gown and gloves (cont.)*

Table 6.4 Summary of ACORN guidelines for gowning and gloving

Gowning	1. Remove the gown from the sterile field and allow it to fall open in front of you. 2. Locate the sleeves and work the arms into them. 3. Keep hands within the sleeves unless the scrub-nurse is to put on your gloves. 4. Allow the back ties of the gown to be tied. 5. Once gloved, spin the wrap-around tie, with other sterile personnel, to cover the back of the gown.
Gloving (closed method)	1. Pick up the left glove, with the right hand, through the sleeve material. 2. Place it palm-to-palm and thumb-to-thumb on the upturned left hand. 3. Grasp the lower fold of the glove, with the left hand, through the sleeve material. 4. Lift the upper fold of the glove over the open sleeve end. 5. Slide the hand into the glove. 6. Repeat on the right hand.
Removing gowns and gloves	1. Undo the wrap-around tie. 2. Allow the back ties to be undone by other staff. 3. Pull down the gown and remove it first, bundle it and deposit in the linen skip. 4. Remove the gloves by grasping the cuffs and turning inside out. 5. Deposit gloves in contaminated disposal bin.

Source: Australian Federation of Operating Room Nurses (ACORN) Standards Manual

amount of contaminant blood removed from a solid needle passing through two layers of latex compared with the same needle passing through just one. Both these advantages of double-gloving *may* reduce the chance of acquiring blood-borne infections from needlestick injuries.

Non-sterile protective equipment, such as masks and eyewear, should be used during procedures and at times of risk from spills, splashes and airborne hazards. The wide variety of masks available are either

Sterile technique

Table 6.5 Surgical gloves

Characteristic	Features
Packaging	Sterile—in sealed packages (for procedures) Clean—in boxes, etc. (for protection)
Material	Latex—most common but allergies Neoprene—for the latex-allergic (staff or patients) Vinyl—as sterile undergloves or non-sterile
Lubricant	Starch—but, remember, granulomas and adhesions may be caused by this substance and it should be avoided if possible None—rely on natural slip to allow gloving
Size	Hand sizes 5½ up to 9 These are standard but tend to vary with manufacturer
Thickness	Variety of thickness—depends on material, manufacturer and the function they are designed for: • special orthopaedic gloves—very thick • micro-thin gloves—for microsurgery. These thinner gloves are easier for double-gloving and don't compromise safety by easier rupture • 'normal'—vary in thickness according to manufacturer and specific material used
Problems	• Allergies to latex • Starch allergies and patient reactions (granulomas and adhesions) • Inconsistencies in manufacture—thickness, holes • Some difficult for double-gloving (esp. no starch) • To guarantee sterility a safe gloving technique (closed method) should be learnt

simple or incorporate a shield (Fig. 6.8). From a philosophical point of view, the facemask is protection as much for the surgeon as the patient. Some studies have suggested that certain types of facemask become saturated within minutes and do not prevent droplets from being blown onto the patient. Despite this, the physical presence of a mask prevents contact between the individual's face and mucous membranes, and powder, aerosols or droplets of body fluids.

Eye protection is an equally important barrier for members of the scrub team. This may be as simple as a shield fitted to a mask, non-prescription glasses with or without side-shields, over-glasses to fit over

Basic Surgical Skills

(a)

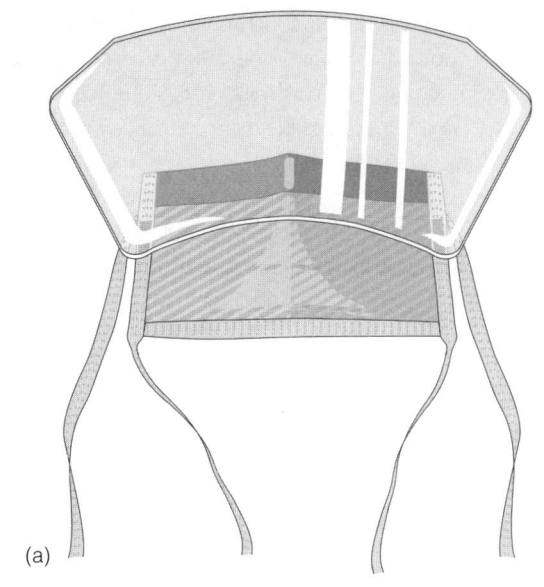

Facemask with attached clear plastic eye shield

(b)

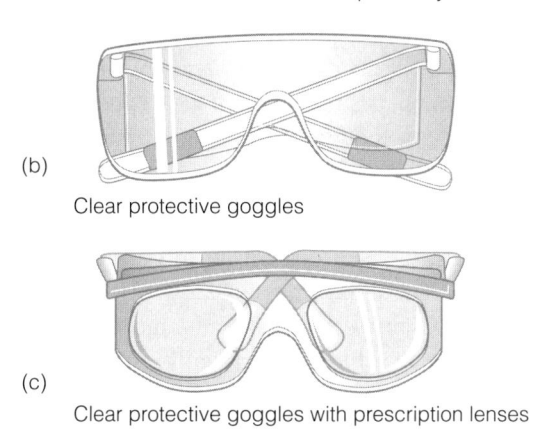

Clear protective goggles

(c)

Clear protective goggles with prescription lenses

Fig. 6.8 *Three types of protective eyewear*

prescription glasses, or even protective frames fitted with prescription lenses.

No-touch technique

This method of operating, used frequently in orthopaedics, involves the use of instruments alone to manipulate and handle tissues, sutures and prostheses. The gloved hand never touches the tissues or any prosthesis inserted into the body. 'No-touch' operating is believed to prevent infections by eliminating the possibility of tissue contact with a glove-borne contamination. Possible sources of this contamination include microscopic breaches in glove material and contact, by the gloves, with the patient's skin or other external source of bacteria. While possible in some specialties, the necessity for tactile impressions and hand dissection makes this technique impractical in others. There is no evidence to suggest that these measures improve patient outcomes in general surgery.

Sterilisation of procedural tools

Sterilisation is the process by which all forms of microbial life (viruses, bacteria, spores and fungi) are completely destroyed. Either a physical or chemical process may achieve this end-point. It is important to recognise that sterility is an absolute concept—that is, an object is either sterile or it is not. *Disinfection*, on the other hand, is a process that destroys all harmful organisms, but not spores, and therefore renders the instrument clean but not sterile. This is usually carried out by soaking the instrument in a disinfectant for a set period of time. Care must be taken to adequately rinse this substance off the instrument, as it may be toxic. Disinfection is not considered further in this section.

Instruments and equipment are sterilised to prevent the spread of infection between consecutive patients on whom items are used, and to patients from the environment. Any instruments whose sterility cannot be guaranteed for any reason must be discarded, resterilised or replaced. Disposable, single-use items come prepacked and sterilised (usually) in ethylene oxide. Most reusable instruments are sterilised in a hospital-based, or regional, Sterile Supply Department. This is usually performed, in bulk, with high-pressure steam methods.

Sterilisation can be undertaken in a number of ways. The first, common step in this process is always the macroscopic removal of debris from the surface of the instrument. This is carried out manually and then the instrument is packed for sterilisation. Steam, dry heat and chemical processes are all used in certain situations. Steam can be used for all wrapped articles (including gowns and drapes) and unwrapped instruments but cannot be used for paper, inks, oils and heat-sensitive items. Dry heat can only be used on anhydrous items that can withstand 160°C for at least one hour. Chemical methods, such as ethylene oxide, can be used for items that cannot tolerate steam or dry methods. Manufacturers, rather than hospital units, may also use ionising radiation to sterilise certain medical devices. A summary can be found in Table 6.7.

Steam sterilisation

Steam is used for the sterilisation of most surgical equipment. The underlying principle of this method is that all microorganisms can be destroyed if their intracellular enzyme/protein systems are denatured and coagulated. Steam, especially when present without other gases, will permeate the packaging of supplies and come into contact with the microorganisms present. Water catalyses these processes and, as the steam condenses to liquid water on the organisms, latent heat is released, fuelling the denaturation and coagulation process. Even spores are destroyed by steam.

At atmospheric pressure, steam exists at a temperature of 100°C and one litre of water produces approximately 860 litres of water vapour. At this temperature steam sterilisation is a very slow process. To increase the steam's temperature the pressure at which it is held must likewise increase. To increase the temperature further any air, which acts as a barrier to the water molecules, must be excluded from the chamber of the steriliser. Increase in pressure and temperature leads to a decrease in time taken for sterilisation (Table 6.6).

Three types of steam steriliser are in common use in hospitals. The traditional autoclave pumps steam into a sealed chamber. The lighter

Table 6.6 International temperature pressure time relationship for steam sterilisation (as outlined in Australian Standard 4187, which specifies the code of practice for sterilising in Australian health-care facilities)

Pressure	Temperature of saturated steam	Holding time at peak temperature required for sterilisation
15 psi / 103 kPa	121°C	15 mins
20 psi / 138 kPa	126°C	10 mins
27 psi / 186 kPa	132°C	3–4 mins

Source: Australian Standard 4187: Code of practice for disinfecting and sterilizing reusable medical and surgical instruments and equipment, and maintenance of associated environments in health care facilities, Standards Australia, Sydney 1994

water vapour displaces the heavier air from the chamber and prevents it mixing with the steam (gravity displacement method). The temperature and pressure are increased by the continued addition of steam to the sealed chamber. Based on the standard requirements (Table 6.6), a sterilising and drying cycle is carried out. All steam-sterilisable material can be processed in an autoclave.

Flash (high-speed) sterilisers are usually gravity displacement in type and are set at 27 psi (186 kPa) and 134°C. Due to the high temperature and pressure, the cycle lasts only for 3–10 minutes. Flash units can be used for most items except implantable prostheses as the reliability of sterilisation may be somewhat reduced due to the speed of the cycle. In most theatre suites, urgently required instruments that are not sterile are the only items to be flash-sterilised.

Prevacuum, high-temperature sterilisers are much faster for routine sterilisation. The air is removed by a pump prior to steam injection into the unit. This means rapid heating occurs and sterilisation time is reduced. Filtered hot air is pumped in at the end of the cycle to dry the contents. In all, this may take as little as 12 minutes to complete.

Dry heat sterilisation

Dry heat sterilisers work on the principle that mechanical convection of dry, hot air, at temperatures of around 160°C, can destroy microorganisms. The cycle must be maintained for one hour at that temperature with extra time required for heating and cooling. Only anhydrous items that cannot be steam-sterilised require this method.

Chemical sterilisation

The use of chemical sterilisation techniques, at low temperatures, is a viable alternative to heat-based sterilisation. The three commonly recognised methods are gas (ethylene oxide), liquid (glutaraldehyde) and plasma (ionised hydrogen peroxide gas).

Gas sterilisation with ethylene oxide takes place at 54–60°C. It requires the presence of some water and is thought to occur by alkylation of cell constituents and prevention of the replication mechanism. Ethylene oxide penetrates most materials, is broadly active, does not require the heat and pressure levels of the other methods and is non-corrosive. However, it is expensive, highly flammable, severely toxic, may be retained in tubular equipment (e.g. tubing) and may damage some plastics. This method should never be used on equipment that can be steam-sterilised.

Liquid sterilisation with a solution of 2% glutaraldehyde is an effective method for certain types of endoscope. Unfortunately, for full sterilisation at least ten hours of soaking is needed. Copious irrigation is required to ensure removal of all toxic chemical.

Plasma sterilisation is a newer method that utilises low-temperature hydrogen peroxide plasma in an hour-long cycle. The sterilising chamber is evacuated of all gas, hydrogen peroxide liquid is introduced and then vaporised. A magnetic or radio-frequency field is then passed through the low pressure gas to ionise the molecules. The reactive cloud of ions, electrons and neutral particles then collides with, and destroys, micro-organisms. It is very effective against all viruses, bacteria, fungi and spores. There is also no toxicity as the ions reconstitute as oxygen or water once they have contacted and killed the organisms present. This method may eventually supersede steam sterilisation.

Conclusions

Sterile technique is the basis for the operative field. Creation and maintenance of this field is one of the skills that must be developed as part of broader surgical training. Intraoperatively, the responsibility for maintaining the field lies with all members of the scrub team. An understanding of all the concepts contained above, including sterilisation procedures, is also essential for the success of the practitioner undertaking any minor surgical procedures.

Further reading

Australian Standard 4187, 'Code of practice for cleaning, disinfecting and sterilizing reusable medical and surgical instruments and equipment, and maintenance of associated environments in health care facilities', Standards Association of Australia, Sydney, 1994.

Friedin J and Marshall V. *Illustrated Guide to Surgical Practice*, Churchill Livingstone, Melbourne, 1984. Chap. 4, The Operation (gowning and gloving).

Gardner JF and Peel MM. *Introduction to Sterilization and Disinfection*, Churchill Livingstone, Melbourne, 1986.

Meeker MH and Rothrock JC (eds). *Alexander's Care of the Patient in Surgery*, 10th edn, Mosby, St Louis, 1995. Chap. 3, Infection Control.

Sterile technique

Table 6.7 Summary of common sterilisation methods

Method	Description	Uses	Precautions
Steam—Autoclave	Air elimination by downward displacement Pressure and temperature dictate cycle (see Table 6.6) Drying component of cycle Microorganism destruction by protein denaturation and coagulation	All loose and wrapped instruments, solutions and drapes that are not temperature-sensitive. Not paper, ink or oil	Pressure vessel precautions and training required Indicators required to confirm efficacy Burns risk
Steam—Flash	Air elimination by downward displacement High pressure and temperature (27 psi / 134°C) Fast cycle with drying component Microorganism destruction by protein denaturation and coagulation	As for autoclave, but should not be used for prostheses. Major user for emergency resterilisation of dropped instruments	As for autoclave Potentially reduced efficacy due to short cycle length
Steam—Vacuum	Rapid air elimination by vacuum extraction Rapid heating to pressure and temperature Drying cycle Speed between autoclave and flash Microorganism destruction by protein denaturation and coagulation	As for autoclave	As for autoclave

Dry heat	Fan-forced hot air Long cycle with heating, sterilising (160°C for 60 mins) and cooling stages Microorganism destruction by drying and heat	For anhydrous, steam-sensitive but heat-resistant articles	Burns risk Indicators required to confirm efficacy
Chemical—Gas	Ethylene oxide / CO_2 mixture with >400mg ethylene oxide per litre, at 36–60°C and 40–100% humidity Shorter cycle times with higher temperatures and gas concentrations (3–7 hours) Microorganism destruction by alkylation and prevention of replication	Temperature- and steam-sensitive articles, especially prostheses in these categories	Major risk of toxicity and flammability of gas requiring environmental monitoring (<0.5 ppm) Plastic corrosion Indicators needed to confirm efficacy
Chemical—Liquid	Glutaraldehyde 2% solution which must be used as a total immersion soak for more than 10 hours to ensure sterilisation	Endoscopes (rarely used)	Patient toxicity with inadequate rinsing
Chemical—Plasma	Vaporised hydrogen peroxide in a vacuum that is ionised by a radio-frequency field Ionised particles strike microorganisms and destroy them	Any steam-sterilisable material as well as temperature- and steam-sensitive articles	Indicators needed to confirm efficacy No toxic effects known ? Harmful effects of radio-frequency field?

Source: Compilation assisted by information from *Alexander's Care of the Patient in Surgery*, 10th edn, Mosby, St Louis 1995; *Australian Standard 4187: Code of practice for disinfecting and sterilizing reusable medical and surgical instruments and equipment, and maintenance of associated environments in health care facilities*, Standards Australia, Sydney 1994; and *Introduction to Sterilization and Disinfection*, Churchill Livingstone, Melbourne 1986

Safety in the operating theatre

In deciding to undertake any invasive procedure, practitioners render themselves vulnerable to the potential hazards of infectious disease, injury and other operating suite dangers. Likewise, the patient and other staff members are exposed to many risks, both related and not related to the procedure. In this chapter these three groups are highlighted and some of the risks inherent in the theatre environment are identified. Strategies for minimisation of these risks are also discussed.

The surgeon and scrub team

This group usually comprises one surgeon, one or two assistants and one scrub-nurse. The major hazards include exposure to body fluids, sharps and other instruments, electricity from equipment used, radiation from x-rays, other equipment risks and, finally, inexperience.

Body substances

Body fluids include blood, urine, pus, gut contents, faeces, pleural fluid, peritoneal fluid, lymph and bile. Other substances such as bone dust and irrigation splash are equally a problem. These may all carry hepatitis B, hepatitis C, other hepatitis viruses and HIV. Avoidance of direct contact or ingestion is the best way to prevent the spread of these conditions. This is most easily facilitated by the strict observance of all barriers (see

Chap. 6) and care with operative technique and tissue handling. It is beyond the scope of this book to discuss the transmission risks of viral and other diseases but there are excellent recent review articles and much other literature on this subject.

The prevention of spills, splashes and other airborne dissemination of substances is a vital safety aspect of surgical technique. Barriers over blood vessels when releasing clamps or checking flow, gentle and careful pouring to avoid spills, not throwing wet or contaminated material, and suction to minimise bone dust when drilling and diathermy smoke when cauterising are all simple measures to reduce the risk.

Sharps and surgical instruments

Sharp surgical instruments are particularly dangerous to the scrub team (see Chap. 2) and special precautions are required for safe handling. The first risk comes with assembly of the scalpel, while attaching the blade to the handle, or removing it at the end of an operation. This procedure should only be undertaken with an instrument (see Fig. 7.1), not with the fingers. Similarly, hollow needles should only be placed onto a syringe while sheathed and should never be resheathed. Suture needles are loaded directly from the packet or handled with forceps.

The process of handing sharps to and from the surgeon is a time of danger for the entire team. All sharps should be passed in a bowl or

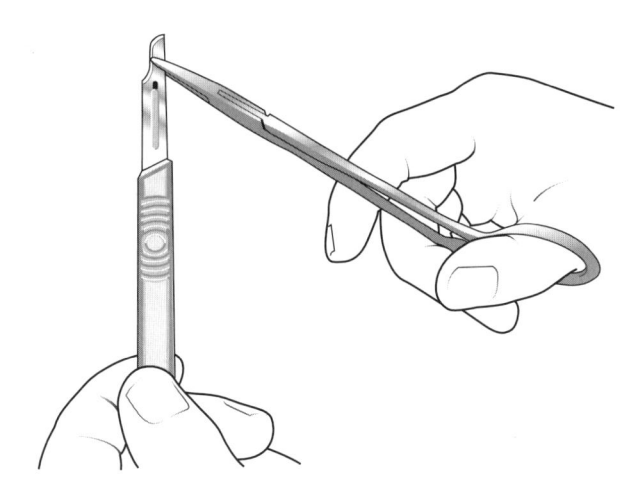

(a) The scalpel blade is inserted onto the handle with an instrument.

Fig. 7.1 *Scalpel blade safety*

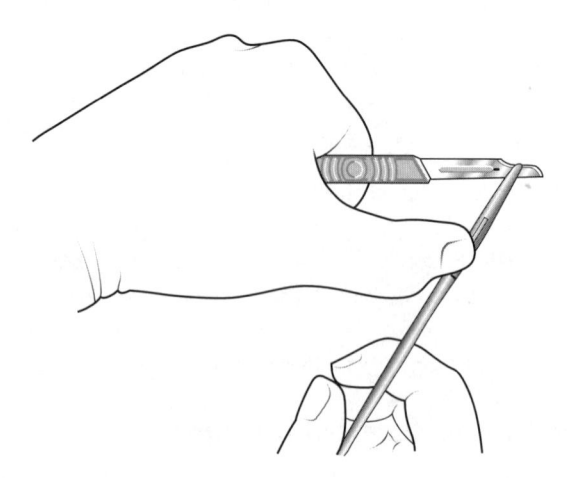

(b) Removing the blade is done with an instrument and is controlled by slowly extending the thumb.

Fig. 7.1 *Scalpel blade safety (cont.)*

kidney dish that is either held by the scrub-nurse or placed in a designated position on the sterile field. It can then be removed and returned with relative safety. The surgeon must concentrate fully on this simple task as inadvertent injury may be caused to other personnel if the movement is made without watching. When finished, if the scrub-nurse is informed that a sharp is returning, the chance of inadvertent injury is probably decreased. When handing back a needle holder the needle should be reversed to protect the point within the jaws of the instrument (see Fig. 2.30). A sharp must never be placed on the patient. It can cut through drapes and injure the patient or any staff members who do not realise it is there.

The basic principle of all instruments, but especially sharps, is that they 'belong' to the scrub-nurse and should be returned to that person while not in use, as this facilitates the maintenance of a safe and uncluttered operative field. Ensure that you return every instrument. They must be counted at the end of the case and it is the scrub-nurse's responsibility to account for and dispose of all sharps (see Table 7.1).

Basic Surgical Skills

> **Table 7.1 Sharps precautions**
>
> - Assemble with care.
> - **Never place a sharp on the patient.**
> - Only ever pass blades, syringes and needles in a dish.
> - When passing a needle holder with needle, protect the point by reversing the needle to point back into the joint of the instrument.
> - Always tell a scrub-nurse that you are passing a sharp back to her.
> - Do not recap sharps.
> - The sharps 'belong' to the scrub-nurse—ensure you return each one as they must be counted at the end of the case.

Other hazards

Radiation and electrical hazards are frequently present in theatre. During the use of x-ray equipment in theatre all personnel within 5 metres of the unit should be shielded by lead. This may be in the form of an apron or screen, or behind a lead-lined wall. Acute exposure is rarely a problem but the cumulative effect of multiple exposures over years is a definite risk factor in the development of various neoplasms.

Electrical hazard, in the form of both micro and macro shock, is constantly present in theatre. The use of monitors, diathermy and various central venous access lines presents risks for both staff and patient. Adequate earthing and special micro-shock electrical safety features make theatre safer but not risk-free.

Care with the use of toxic substances is also vital as these are often found in theatre. Glutaraldehyde, a disinfectant for endoscopes, formalin, a preservative in specimen bottles, and many toxic cleaning chemicals are included on this list. To protect staff, careful handling of the substances, minimisation of handling and special equipment or ventilated work spaces are all required.

The final factor, inexperience, can exacerbate any of the preceding potential risk factors. In not understanding the general principles, specific practices and the 'flow' of theatre, the novice may unintentionally cause harm. Adequate pre-theatre instruction in these areas combined with some 'bench-training' in both safety and surgical techniques seems, intuitively, to be one way of minimising the effect of practical inexperience.

Universal Precautions

The concept that all body substances may carry transmissible agents, no matter how 'safe' the patient appears, has led to the development of a set of Universal Precautions. These guidelines for safe patient contact put a physical barrier between all patients, their attendant health workers and other patients, thereby preventing the spread of diseases in either direction. Without exception the precautions should be used with all patients, in all situations. Hand washing, the use of barriers (gowns/gloves/glasses/masks) and the safe disposal of sharp or contaminated materials are the cornerstones of this practice.

To put these precautions into practice in theatre is quite simple. First, hands are washed with antimicrobial soap before each procedure. Generally, all members of the scrub team wear masks, eye protection, sterile gowns and sterile gloves. These prevent direct contact with body substances and preserve sterility in direct contacts with the patient. Further to these basic precautions, gowns may be made from waterproof material, or a plastic apron can be worn under a cloth gown to prevent contact from 'soak through'.

Gloves can also be worn double (there are now micro-thin options) to prevent skin–fluid contact despite holing one or both layers. Unfortunately, this practice does not prevent needlesticks or penetrating injuries from other instruments.

The patient

There are three distinct phases during the transit of any procedural patient through hospital and each has different inherent risks. These phases can be broadly defined as preparation for the procedure, the procedure itself and the post-procedure period. At any stage in this cycle, patients are at risk from both the environment of the operating suite and the effects of the procedures they undergo.

Preparation for the procedure

Prior to commencing a procedure it is essential for each patient to be adequately prepared. This entails appropriate patient education, necessary paperwork and indicated investigations. The patient must then be transferred to the theatre suite. Once in theatre, transfer to the operating table, anaesthesia and correct positioning are undertaken.

It is essential to ensure that the correct patient is being operated on and that the patient is fit for the procedure. A consent form should be signed detailing the correct site of operation and the correct side, and the patient should understand both the procedure and its risks. Optimally, the lesion should be marked to avoid intraoperative confusion, and all x-rays and test results must be available in theatre. Allergies, drug reactions and special patient precautions should also be detailed preoperatively. These measures will minimise simple errors such as amputating the right leg instead of the left (see Table 7.2).

Table 7.2   Preoperative precautions for the patient

- The correct patient is being operated on and is fit for the procedure.
- Consent is signed, the correct site and side are on it and the patient understands both the procedure and its risks.
- The correct organ/system/limb is being operated on.
- The correct side is being operated on.
- The lesion is marked to avoid intraoperative confusion.
- All x-rays and test results are available in theatre.
- Allergies, drug reactions and special patient precautions are known.

Once in theatre the patient must be moved from the trolley or bed to the operating table. The patient may be able to move himself, but this is fraught with danger. Premedicated patients can be unreliable at this and, if wheels on either the bed or table are not locked, one of them may move, leaving a gap for the patient to fall through. Alternative methods of moving the patient include the use of poles through a canvas undersheet or lifting the patient directly. Both these methods, however, can strain the back of the lifter. Various roller and smooth polycarbonate sliding boards have been developed to facilitate sliding the patient from a higher surface to a lower, and these are now the most common option.

Once on the operating table the patient must be positioned for easy access to the operative site. This is facilitated by being able to 'bend' the table at various points (called 'breaking the table'), roll the table and insert bolsters or beanbags to stabilise the patient. Armboards may be used to support one or both arms and greatly improve access to drips, arterial lines and other monitoring equipment. In general, positioning is supervised by the surgeon with the assistance of technicians and other available staff. Theatre technicians are trained in this art and junior doctors should usually only assist with the process, rather than try to direct it.

Before moving an anaesthetised patient the anaesthetist should secure the endotracheal tube in position and check that all drips and other lines are not going to tangle during the move. Hasty movement of the patient may result in the pulling out of lines or even injury to the patient from this or other mishaps.

No matter what position the patient is in, certain precautions must be observed. There must be no metal-to-skin contact in order to prevent diathermy burns from accidental earthing of the patient. Any pressure on bony prominences and nerves must be avoided or padded to prevent injury. Abnormal traction or angulation of limbs or neck must be prevented or joint, bone and nerve injuries may occur. All anaesthetised patients' eyes should be taped shut to prevent drying. Some form of deep venous thrombosis (DVT) prophylaxis should be used in cases longer than half an hour, in the elderly, in patients with a past history of DVT or with any risk factor for deep venous thrombosis. Finally, if there is any risk of patient movement on the table, sets of padded retaining bolsters and strong adhesive taping should be used to prevent this (see Table 7.3).

Table 7.3 Precautions needed when positioning the patient

- There must be no metal-to-skin contact in order to prevent diathermy burns from accidental earthing of the patient.
- Pressure on bony prominences and nerves must be avoided or padded to prevent injury.
- Abnormal traction or angulation must be avoided.
- Eyes should be taped shut to prevent drying.
- DVT prophylaxis should be used in cases longer than half an hour, in the elderly, in patients with a past history of DVT and patients with any other risk factor.
- If there is any risk of patient movement, padded retaining bolsters and taping should be used to prevent this.

The operative site should then be prepared with an antiseptic substance to which the patient is not allergic. All alcoholic preparations should be allowed to dry prior to the use of diathermy, because of the fire risk. Any type of tourniquet must have a time limit set before its application. Inflation or application time, and deflation or removal time should be recorded in the patient's chart. These precautions should prevent lengthy ischaemia or failure to remove the tourniquet.

The procedure

During any procedure there are multiple potential hazards to the patient. These are usually the adverse effects of routine equipment usage or procedure itself. Occasionally they are due to the actions or errors of a member of the scrub team.

Instruments have significant potential for harming a patient. Incorrect or careless use of scalpels, scissors or any instrument with a sharp edge may result in damage to adjacent structures, and overly vigorous use of a retractor may result in contusion or frank injury such as ruptured spleen, liver or bowel. Use of instruments should be adequately explained to the inexperienced and unfamiliar assistant or trainee, and you should not hesitate to request a demonstration if unsure of the correct technique of use.

Other equipment such as diathermy (see Chap. 2), anaesthetic equipment, tourniquets, lasers, endoscopes and gauzes all have their own problems. Essentially, like surgical instruments, adequate training in their use will eliminate many of these risks. Sterile technique can itself be a problem. Inadvertent breaches in technique, combined with the presumption of absolute sterility, may result in infective complications for the patient. Any suspected breach in sterility, then, must be dealt with promptly and completely for the benefit of the patient (see Table 7.4).

After the procedure

Even when a procedure is complete the patient is still at risk as this period contains many hazards applicable to the procedure itself. Transfer from the procedure table has the same risks as transferring on but compounded by the level of anaesthesia. Accidental dislodgement of tubes or drips is not uncommon and must be prevented by vigilance prior to the move. Potential injuries to the patient because of his level of anaesthesia include fractures and dislocations (even of the spine), lacerations and even 'dropping' the patient if the bed and table move apart. Such incidents are inexcusable and often reflect poor planning, haste, lack of experience and inadequate numbers of staff.

While recovering from the anaesthetic there are risks of airway compromise and effects of the drugs that have been administered. A very high nurse/patient ratio in the Post-Anaesthesia Care Unit (PACU) reflects

Table 7.4 Hazards of the equipment

Equipment	Hazard
Sharps	Needlestick injury
	Accidental laceration and trauma to adjacent structures
	Inadvertent division of, or damage to, structures
Retractors	Toe damage deep within the abdomen and chest
	Skin bruising
	Traction injuries to nerves or vessels
Forceps	Puncture wounds
	Tearing of structures
Sutures	Tear out and damage tissues
	Puncture viscera (needle)
	Knots unwind and reduce wound strength
	May provide a nidus for infection
Diathermy	Flux injuries and direct contact accidents
	Electrocution
	Burns to the surgeon
	Inadvertent division of, or damage to, structures
Gauze/Packs	May be left inside the patient by accident
	Wipes off clots, causing bleeding
Suckers	Promotes bleeding by vigorous suction
	Traumatises tissues

the need for close observation. Post-anaesthetic observations are carried out to assess the patient's airway, cardiorespiratory status, conscious state and level of pain relief. It is only once the patient is awake, stable and comfortable that he will be transferred back to the ward.

For the PACU to be a source of complications is uncommon but it can certainly be the area in which they are detected. The incorrect administration of drugs, incorrect connection of breathing circuits and electrical equipment faults are some of the ways in which PACU may actually cause the problem.

Other personnel

Common-sense attitudes are required to ensure safety for other theatre staff. All efforts must be made to prevent spills of blood and other body fluids. Only a fully gowned and gloved member of the scrub team should deal with soiled drapes or instruments, and assistance should be provided with lifting/sliding the patient to reduce the strain on each person. These are just a few examples of how a mutually supportive, team approach to tasks will benefit the whole theatre with little inconvenience to the individual.

A pleasant and helpful demeanour, while frequently derided, will usually ensure that good relations are maintained with theatre staff. This will make all processes smoother and improve work satisfaction for all. Remember, while medical staff must bear the greatest responsibility in regard to theatre procedures, we are all members of a health-care team dedicated to just one thing—the optimum care of a patient.

Glossary

Some definitions in this glossary were compiled with the assistance of *Butterworths Medical Dictionary*, 2nd edn, Butterworths, London 1978

abrasion Removal of part of the skin by rubbing (graze).

absorption The taking in of a material passively by a semi-solid substance, or actively by a body through its alimentary or vascular systems.

action potential Localised depolarisation and repolarisation of the cell membrane in a segment of an excitable tissue, which is propagated along or through that tissue.

adrenaline Vasoactive substance released from the adrenal medulla and also chemically manufactured. May be added to local anaesthetics and is a potent vasoconstrictor when injected locally.

allergic reaction Local or generalised body response to an antigen that usually involves an inflammatory reaction and, sometimes, tissue damage. *Synonym:* hypersensitivity reaction.

allergy See **allergic reaction**.

anaemia Reduction in erythrocyte numbers and/or haemoglobin concentration in the blood.

Basic Surgical Skills

antigen Substance that may stimulate a hypersensitivity (allergic) reaction.

antiseptic Substance able to destroy harmful organisms in a tissue but sufficiently non-toxic to allow application to the tissue.

aseptic Free from infection or pathogenic organisms.

bend A turn or angle in a knot.

blunt dissection The process of opening fascial planes by splitting, stripping, squeezing, teasing or pulling. May be effected by instruments or fingers.

bow The finger rings of an instrument.

brachial plexus Plexus of cervical and upper thoracic nerves that supplies the upper limb. Begins in the supraclavicular fossa and extends into the axilla.

burn Injury to tissue caused by heat, cold or chemicals.

cell membrane The lipid bilayer which surrounds all cells. Comprises two layers of molecules which have an outer lipophilic segment and an inner hydrophilic segment that interacts with the hydrophilic segment of opposing molecules.

chilblain Peripheral inflammatory lesion caused by exposure to cold.

collagen Amorphous glycine and proline rich substance, mainly white in colour, found abundantly in bone, tendons and connective tissue.

collagenolysis The breakdown of collagen, at the wound edge, by collagenase enzymes.

compartment syndrome Raised pressure in a fascial bound compartment (e.g. forearm) leading to reduced tissue perfusion pressures and consequent ischaemic damage to tissues within the compartment. Occurs before blood flow in major vessels passing through the compartment is compromised.

concussion Post-head-injury state characterised by brief loss of consciousness, transient confusion, amnesia and headache.

contre-coup Damage to the brain occurring diametrically opposite the site of trauma to the skull.

contusion Superficial bruising injury without a break in the skin.

counter-traction The process of putting tension on tissues to be divided.

CPR Cardiopulmonary resuscitation.

CSF Cerebrospinal fluid.

cyanosis Bluish tissue colour caused by the presence of deoxygenated haemoglobin.

debridement The process of removing foreign bodies and dead and devitalised tissue from a wound to allow healing to occur more rapidly and without infection.

delayed primary closure Closing a wound by initially not closing the skin and then subsequently bringing the edges together, with any method, at a time significantly removed (> 1 day) from the time it was first surgically created or treated.

depilation Removal of hair.

depolarisation The process where an actively maintained, negative resting potential (polarisation) across a membrane is returned towards neutrality by the influx, through electrically opened channels, of positive ions (sodium) into the cell.

diathermy Electrosurgical instrument used for cutting and haemostasis.

diathermy, bipolar Diathermy where the two active electrodes are the tips of a pair of forceps and current flows only between these points. Used when current flow at the point required would be dangerous, e.g. brain, digits, penis.

diathermy, monopolar Diathermy where one active electrode is the tip of an instrument and the other is a gel pad attached to the patient. The patient then becomes part of the diathermy circuit as opposed to bipolar diathermy when they do not.

disinfect The process of removing pathogenic organisms.

dissection The process of dividing tissues to display an organ or structure.

drapes Sterile sheets used to maintain the sterile operative field.

ductility   The ability to be drawn out to form a wire; refers specifically to metals.

ecchymosis   Small haematoma arising on the site of a bruise.

elasticity   The ability to recover an original size and shape after any sort of distortion.

EMST   Early Management of Severe Trauma course developed by the RACS and based on the American Advanced Trauma Life Support (ATLS) course. Provides a reproducible and safe framework for trauma management based on the principle of excluding all potential injuries.

epithelium   Closely packed cells, arranged in layers, which cover the body surface and all the tubular structures that open on the surface (e.g. GI tract, urinary tract).

eschar   Thickened slough of necrotic skin and subcutaneous tissue in the area of a burn.

excitable tissues   Tissues able to be stimulated to depolarise and conduct electrical impulses, e.g. muscle and nerve.

exposure   Displaying tissues to be operated upon by the division or excision of other tissues more superficially placed.

fascia   Connective tissues of all types.

fascial planes/tissue planes   Planes of cleavage between structures, organs and other fascia held together (usually) with areolar connective tissue.

fibroblast   Common, spindle-shaped, connective tissue cell which produces collagen.

first intention healing   Healing, by granulation and fibrosis, of the closely opposed edges of a wound.

following   Holding suture threads out of the way while a continuous suture is performed, 40% of the thread on the assistant's side of the grip and 60% on the surgeon's.

forcep   Grasping instrument.

frostbite   Tissue injury caused by partial or complete freezing of the water in cells of the affected part.

granulation tissue   The loops of ingrowing capillaries, and their bed of collagen, cells and ground substance, which leads to the healing of all wounds.

haemostasis   The prevention and arrest of bleeding by procedural means.

hydro-dissection   The process of improving tissue planes for dissection by the injection of fluid. May be intentional or a happy side effect of local anaesthetic use.

hydrolysis   The splitting of a molecule by the addition of water which in turn supplies a hydrogen and a peroxide ion to bind with the free ends of the break.

hypersensitivity   An excessive host reaction to an antigen which the host has previously been sensitised to.

hypotension   Low blood pressure, usually below 100 mmHg systolic.

hypoxia   Reduced arterial oxygen to the tissues resulting in an inability to maintain aerobic metabolism.

immersion foot   Similar injury to trenchfoot but longer exposure to warmer water is the initiating factor. Develops over weeks to months.

incised wound   Traumatic wound created by a sharp-edged object.

incision   Linear cut made by a sharp-edged instrument or object.

infection   The invasion of the body by pathogenic organisms and their subsequent multiplication.

insufflation   The process of inflating a body or organ cavity with gas (usually carbon dioxide or air) for the process of endoscopy.

intramuscular   Within a muscle.

intravenous   Into a vein.

laceration   Ragged and untidy wound made by the tearing of tissues with a sharp or blunt object.

laparoscope   Endoscopic instrument for examining the peritoneal cavity.

ligating   Securing with a length of thread tied around the structure in question.

local anaesthetic Substance that inhibits nerve cell depolarisation and hence numbs the region supplied by the sensory fibres of the nerve. Also has a motor effect.

malnutrition Faulty nutrition due to an inadequate supply, or absorption, of food.

membrane pumps Membrane-bound channels through which substances are actively transported by a carrier system requiring energy to function.

membrane stabilisation The prevention of membrane depolarisation by a substance that inhibits the function of passive ion channels, e.g. a local anaesthetic.

mobilisation The process of freeing an organ from natural and acquired (adhesional) tissue attachments to make it easier to work on, or to reveal structures it may obscure.

myofibroblast Fibroblast with contractile properties that aids in wound contraction.

needle holder Forcep designed specifically to hold a needle and drive it through tissue.

neurone Nerve cell.

nylon Synthetic material developed by DuPont chemicals, during the 1940s, in their New York (Ny-) and London (-lon) laboratories.

PACU Post-anaesthetic care unit.

phagocytosis The process of ingestion of dead or foreign material by specific white blood cells.

prep and drape Process of preparing the skin of the operative site with a disinfectant solution and placing drapes to define the operative field and the sterile area.

primary closure Closing a wound by bringing the edges together with any method, at the time it is first surgically created or treated.

proteolysis The breakdown of protein, by hydrolysis, into soluble degradation products.

pseudocholinesterase Enzymes of the cholinesterase family that split the choline esters (such as succinylcholine) but not acetylcholine.

pus Liquid product of inflammation containing dead white blood cells, tissue and bacteria (if infective).

pyogenic Pus producing.

pyrogenic Fever producing.

RACS Royal Australasian College of Surgeons.

receptor 1. Specialised nerve ending that detects a specific stimulus. 2. Specialised molecular grouping in a cell membrane that detects a specific substance or group of substances.

repolarisation The return of a cell membrane to the polarised state after the passage of an excitatory impulse.

retraction The act of drawing away superficial tissues to facilitate the intraoperative display of structures.

retractor Instrument designed specifically to hold tissue aside in the operative field. May be hand-held or self-retaining.

reverse contamination Contamination of staff by body substances released by the sterile operative field, e.g. blood, pus or faeces.

rigidity Stiffness or inflexibility.

scald Superficial burn caused by liquid or vapour.

scalpel Bladed cutting instrument. May be reusable or disposable, and one- or two-piece.

second intention healing Healing by granulation, contraction, fibrosis and re-epithelialisation in an open wound or ulcer.

septicaemia Blood-borne infection.

sharp dissection The process of dividing tissues with a sharp instrument such as a knife or scissors.

shock State of inadequate tissue perfusion leading to tissue-level hypoxia, anaerobic metabolism and subsequent (lactic) acidosis.

simple suture The basic semi-circular suture upon which all others are based.

skin Epidermis and dermis complex.

sterile Free from all microorganisms.

sterile field   All parts of the operation site covered in preparation solution or sterile (green) drapes.

subcutaneous   Below the skin (usually a layer of adipose tissue).

suture   1. A surgical stitch. 2. The act of inserting a surgical stitch. 3. The thread used in a surgical stitch. 4. The interlocking joins between cranial bones.

synapse   The microscopic region where two neurones virtually touch. Within a synapse there is active release of neurotransmitters from one side which are detected by receptors on the other side of the gap. This process propagates the action potential from one neurone to the next.

tension   The pull of tissues against each other. Desirable when incising or dissecting but harmful if present in sutured wounds and anastomoses as it will predispose to wound failure.

threshold potential   The level of polarisation at which ion channels open and the cell membrane depolarises.

toxicity   The level of damage or noxious reaction that a substance, or organism, will produce in living tissues.

trenchfoot   Cold injury to the peripheries (usually feet) caused by immersion for long periods (days to weeks) in near freezing water.

Universal Precautions   A set of standard barriers that are used with every patient to prevent the contamination of staff and other patients by bodily fluids.

Index

abdominal incision, 161, 163
abrasion, 220
absorption, 220
action potential, 220
adrenaline, 36, 154, 181, 220
allergic reaction, 220
anaemia, 30, 220
anaesthesia, 36, 113
anaesthetics, local, 171, 225
    administration, 181
        cavity infusion, 175, 183
        centrineural block, 175, 183
        intravenous (Bier's) block, 174, 179, 182
        local infiltration, 174, 181
            see also local infiltration anaesthesia
        nerve blockade, 174, 182
        topical anaesthesia, 174, 181
    amides, 176
    complications, 178–81
    contraindications, 179, 180
    dosages, 176
    esters, 176
    mechanism of action, 171–3
    precautions, 179, 180
    reactions, 178
    toxicity, 178, 179–81
    uses, 173–5
anaesthetist, 115
analgesia, 183
anatomy, 116, 158
antibiotics, 35
    cephalexin, 35
    dicloxacillin, 35
    erythromycin, 35
    flucloxacillin, 35
    gentamicin, 35
    metronidazole, 35
    penicillin V, 35
antigen, 221
antimicrobial solutions, 113–14
antiseptic, 221
arterial tourniquet, 154, 156
artery forceps, 60, 61, 62–4, 154
asepsis, 187, 221
aspirin, 154
assistant, 113, 116, 163–4
assisting at operation, 116, 163
    exposure, 163, 164
    following, 167–8
    haemostasis, 169
    incisions, 165
    insertion of catheters, 165
    postoperative, 170
    preoperative, 164–5
    retraction, 164, 165–6
    skin stapling, 169
    tension, 166–7
    tying/suture skills, 168–9
    wound closure, 169
Australian Confederation of Operating Room Nurses (ACORN)
    gowning/gloving guidelines, 201
    surgical scrub guidelines, 193
autoclaves, 205–6, 208

bandage sizes, 39
Bier's block, 174, 179, 182
bleeding, 29, 153
    arterial, 115, 157
    capillary oozing, 89, 157–8
    clamps, 156
    diathermy, 154, 157
    excessive, 116
    management, 153, 158
    pressure, 156–7
    prevention, 153–8
    slings, 156, 157
    tamponade, 158
    venous, 157–8
blood vessels see vessels
blood–brain barrier, 114
blunt dissection, 158, 159–62, 221
blunt injury, 6–10, 12, 18
body substances, 210–11
bone cutters, 50–1
bone nibblers, 50–1
bowel, 71, 72
bowel clamps, 71
    crushing, 72
    Doyen, 71
    Lang–Stevenson, 72
    non-crushing, 71
    Parker–Kerr, 72
bowls, 86, 87
bows, 221
brachial plexus, 221
brain injury, 6
bupivicaine, 177
burns, 16, 221
    classification, 16–17
    first-degree, 16, 17, 20
    genital, 18
    ocular, 18
    respiratory, 18
    rule of nines, 18, 19
    second-degree, 16, 17, 20
    thickness, 17
    third-degree (full thickness), 16–18, 20

carbolic acid, 187
catgut, 100, 102–4, 118
cavitation, 10, 15
cavity infusion analgesia, 175, 183
cell death, 24
cell membrane, 221

Index

centrineural blocks, 175, 183
cephalexin, 35
chemical injury, 6, 13, 21, 23
chilblains, 16, 18, 22, 221
chlorhexidine, 37, 191
clamps
    bowel, 71–2
    vascular, 60–1, 62, 65–6, 156
Clostridium tetani, 36
closure, of wounds, 38, 169
    assessment of need, 33, 35
clotting, 153–4
coagulation, 86, 90, 158
coagulopathy, 153
cold injury, 12–13, 16, 18–19, 21, 22
    chilblains, 16, 18, 22
    frostbite, 16, 19, 21, 22
    trenchfoot, 16, 18, 22
collagen, 26, 27, 221
collagenolysis, 29, 221
communication, 35
compartment syndrome, 18, 23, 221
concussion, 221
consent form, 215
containers, 86, 87
contamination, 194
    macroscopic, 191
    reverse, 187, 188, 226
contre-coup brain injury, 6, 8, 221
contusion, 222
counter-traction, 222
curettes, 52
current density, 87–8, 89
cutting instruments, 41
    bone cutters, 50–1
    bone nibblers, 50–1
    curettes, 52
    periosteal elevator, 51–2
    scalpels, 41–2
        blades, 41, 43
        handles, 42
    scissors *see* scissors
    skin graft knives, 49–50
        Humby Knife, 50
        Silver knife, 50
cyanosis, 115, 222

de-epithelialisation, 16
debridement, 26, 37, 149–53, 222
deceleration, of body, 6, 9–10
deep venous thrombosis (DVT)
    prophylaxis, 216
delayed primary closure, 25, 38, 222
delipidation, 21
depilation, 222
depolarisation, 222
dermatome, 49
diathermy, 86–8, 114, 222
    argon beam, 89
    bipolar, 86–7, 88, 90, 222
    bleeding, 154, 157
    current density, 87–8, 89
    monopolar, 86, 87, 88–90, 163, 222
        coagulation mode, 90, 163
        cut mode, 89–90, 163
dicloxacillin, 35
disinfection, 204, 222
dissection, 158–9, 222
    blunt, 158, 159–62
    finger fracture, 161

    pinching, 160–1
    sharp, 158, 162–3
    splitting technique, 161–2
    tension, 159, 162
double-gloving, 198, 201, 214
drapes, 114, 191, 222
draping, 193–4
    shut-out draping, 194, 196, 197
    square draping, 194, 196
duck-billed vaginal speculum, 80
ductility, 223

ecchymosis, 223
elasticity, 223
electrical injury, 6, 13, 23
energy transfer, 6, 7
epithelialisation, 16
epithelium, 223
equipment
    clean, in theatre, 191
    hazards to patient, 217, 218
    protective, 201–3
erythromycin, 35
eschar, 223
escharotomy, 18
excision, 144–9, 158
    skin lesion (example), 146–8
exposure, of tissues, 164, 165–6, 167, 223
eye protection, 201, 202–3

facemasks, 201–2
fascia, 223
fascial planes, 223
fasciotomy, 18
fibroblast, 223
finger fracture dissection technique, 161
first intention healing, 24–5, 27, 38, 223
flucloxacillin, 35
following, 167–8, 223
forceps, 53, 223
    Adson, 55–6, 117
    Allis, 59, 60
    artery, 60, 61, 62–4
        curved, 63
        straight, 63
    Babcock, 59, 61
    Bulldog, vascular clamp, 62
    Debakey
        atraumatic, 57, 58
        vascular clamp, 62
    dissecting, 54, 58
    dressing, 57, 58
    Duvall, 59, 61
    gall-bladder, 72–3
    Gillies, 56, 117
    Halsted, 63
    Kocher's, 59, 63, 64, 72
    Lahey, 73–4
    Lane's
        hand-held, 56
        ratcheted, 59, 60
    McIndoe, 57
    Mixter, 73–4
    Mosquito, 61, 63
    Moynihan, 72–3
    needle-holding, 66–70
    non-toothed, 57, 58
    packing, 58
    Rampley's, sponge-holding, 72, 74, 75
    right-angled, 73–4
    Roberts, long, 61, 63

Index

Rutherford-Morrison, 59, 60
skin-hook, 117
Spencer-Wells, 61, 63
tissue forceps, 60
    hand-held (thumb), 53–4, 55–8
    ratcheted (scissor-style), 53, 54–5, 59–60
    vascular, 60–2
        crushing (haemostatic), 60–1
        non-crushing, 60, 62
fractures, 6, 33
    skull, 8
    tibia, 9, 10
frostbite, 16, 19, 22, 223
    levels of severity, 19, 21
fulguration, 89

gallipot, 87
gangrene, 2, 18, 36
gas exposure, 23
gas sterilisation, 204–5, 206–7, 209
gentamicin, 35
gloves, 197–8
    features, 202
    removing, 201
gloving, 200, 201
    double-gloving, 198, 201, 214
gowning, 199, 201
gowns, 197, 198, 214
    removing, 201
granulation, 38
granulation tissue, 26, 27, 224
grasping instruments, 53
    bowel clamps, 71–2
    gall-bladder forceps, 72–3
    needle-holding forceps, 66–70
        locking, 68–70
        non-locking, 70
    right-angled forceps, 73–4
    sponge-holding forceps, 72, 74, 75
    tissue forceps, 53
        hand-held (or thumb) forcep, 53–4, 55–8
        scissor pattern (ratcheted), 53, 54–5, 59–60
    vascular clamps/forceps
        crushing (haemostatic), 60–1
        non-crushing, 60, 62, 65–6

haematoma, 29, 118, 156
haemostasis, 37, 89, 153–8, 169, 224
headlight, 113
healing see wound healing
heat liberation, 21
heat sterilisation, 204, 206, 209
hydro-dissection, 224
hydrolysis, 224
hyperextension, 9, 11
hyperflexion, 9, 11
hyperkalaemia, 23
hypersensitivity, 224
    see also allergic reaction
hypotension, 224
hypoxia, 224

immersion foot, 18, 224
incisions, 144–9, 224
    diathermy, 145
    Lanz, 161–2
    laparotomy, 148–9
    marking, 144

infection, 2, 18, 29, 118, 224
instruments, 40
    bows, 221
    hazards, 211–12
    palming, 45, 54, 68, 69
    placement in theatre, 113–14
    see also cutting instruments; grasping instruments; retractors
insufflation, 224
ionising radiation injury, 13, 23–4
irradiation, 30
ischaemia, 18, 28, 116, 118, 122

jaundiced patients, 153
    vitamin K, 153

kidney dishes, 86, 87
kinetic energy (blunt) injury, 6–10, 12
kinetic energy (penetrating) injury, 6, 10, 12, 14–15
knot tying, 130–1
    instrument-tied knot, 131, 132–6
    one-handed knot, 131, 136–44
    two-handed knot, 131, 144
knots, 130
    bend, 221
    flat, laid-down, 131
    granny knot, 130
    half-hitch, 130, 131
    reef knot, 130
    sliding hitch, 131
    surgeon's knot, 130, 131

laceration, 224
    stellate, 6, 7
laminar airflow, 190
laparoscope, 224
ligating, 91, 224
light, operating, 113
lignocaine, 177
liquefaction, 21
Lister, Joseph, 187
local anaesthetic see anaesthetics, local
local infiltration anaesthesia, 181, 184
    aspiration, 184
    dilution, 184
    infiltration technique, 184–5
    needle, 184
    pressure on site, 185
    timing, 184

malnutrition, 225
masks, protective, 201–2
mechanism of injury, 6–24
membrane pumps, 225
membrane stabilisation, 173, 225
metronidazole, 35
mobilisation, 225
myofibroblasts, 26–7, 225
myoglobinuria, 23

necrotising fasciitis, 36
needle holders see needle-holding forceps
needle-holding forceps, 66–70, 225
    Crile-Wood, 70
    Gillies, 70
    holding, 68
    jaws, 66, 67
    locking, 68–70
    Macphail, 67

Index

Mayo-Hegar, 67, 68, 70
Olsen-Hegar, 70
palming techniques, 68, 69
protection of needle point, 69
Ryder, vascular, 67, 70
needles, 40, 91, 92–7
  body, 95, 96
  chord length, 92, 93
  curvature, 92, 93
  curved, 94
  diameter, 92, 93
  eyed, 91, 95, 97
  J-shaped, 93, 94
  length, 92, 93–4
  point, 92, 93, 96
  radius, 92, 93
  shape, 94
  swaged, 91, 92, 93, 95–7
  types
    blunt, 94, 95
    cutting (conventional), 94–5, 117
    reverse cutting, 94, 95, 117
    taper, 94, 95, 117
nerve blockade, 174, 182
nerve depolarisation, 172–3
neurone, 225
no-touch technique, 203–4
nylon, 99, 225

ocular injuries
  burn, 18
  chemical, 23
operating skills see surgical skills
operative field, 112–13
  draping, 113, 114
  instruments, 114–15
  lighting, 113
  maintenance, 113
  preparation, 113–14, 216
  sterile areas, 192

palming, 45
  forceps, 54
  needle holders, 68, 69
penetrating wounds, 6, 12, 14–15, 18
  high-velocity, 10, 12
  low-velocity, 10, 12, 14
penicillin V, 35
periosteal elevator, 51–2
pernio, 18
phagocytosis, 225
poliglecaprone 25, 106
polydioxanone, 101, 105
polyglactin 910, 104–5
polyglycolic acid (PGA), 104
Post-Anaesthesia Care Unit (PACU), 217–18
povidone-iodine, 37, 191
prep and drape, 225
prep solutions, 114, 192–3, 195
  alcohol-based, 37, 114, 163, 193
pressure garments, 16, 18
prilocaine, 177
primary wound closure, 2, 24–5, 225
  delayed, 25, 38, 222
proteolysis, 225
pseudocholinesterase, 225
pus, 226

radiation injury, 6, 13, 23–4
re-epithelialisation, 16, 27
receptors, defined, 226

renal failure, 23
repolarisation, 226
resting tremor, 113
retraction, 74, 226
retractors, 74, 226
  Balfour-Doyen, 81, 82
  cats-paw, 75–6
  crank, 81, 83
  Czerny, 77
  Deaver, 78, 79
  Denis Browne ring, 84
  Durham-Barr, 77
  Finichetto, 81, 83
  Fritsch, 77, 78
  hand-held, 75–8
  hook, 83
  Joll thyroid, 80, 81
  Kelly, 78
  Kocher, 77
  Langenbeck, 77
  lighted, 113
  Morris, 77
  rake, 75–6
  ratcheted, 79, 80
  screw-thread, 79, 80, 81
  self-retaining, 78–83
  skin-hook, 75–6
  spring, 79–80
  St Mark's pelvic, 78, 79
  toe-in movement, 75, 76
  upper-hand, 81, 82
  Weitlaner, 80
reverse contamination, 187, 188, 226
rigidity, 226
ropivicaine, 177

safety, in theatre, 210
  body substance hazards, 210–11
  electrical hazards, 213
  inexperience, 213
  instrument hazards, 211–12
  patient, 214
    equipment hazards, 217, 218
    positioning, 215–16
    post-anaesthesia hazards, 217–18
    precautions, 215, 216
    preparation for theatre, 214–15
    transfers, 215, 217, 219
  radiation risks, 213
  sharps handling, 211–13
  theatre staff, 218–19
  toxic substances, 213
  Universal Precautions, 214
scalds, 16, 226
scalpels, 144, 162, 226
  blades, 41, 43
    blade safety, 211–12
  cutting rules, 42, 149
  handles, 42
  pen grip, 42, 144, 145
  underhand grip (dinner knife), 41, 144, 145, 149
scar, fine and linear, 37
scarring, 16, 18, 24, 27, 100
scissors, 43–4
  angled, 48–9
  curved, 44, 46, 47
  dissecting, 45, 46–7, 162–3
  dressing, 48
  Dubois, 46, 47
  Ferguson's, 48

Index

Golighers, 46
handling, 44–5
Mayo, 46, 47, 48
Metzenbaum, 46
Nurses', 48
Pott's, 48–9
suture, 48
vascular, 48–9
scrub nurse, 114–15, 164, 212
scrub team, 218–19
second intention healing, 25, 26–7, 226
septicaemia, 226
sharp dissection, 158, 162–3, 226
sharps
   'owned' by scrub nurse, 212
   safe handling, 211–13
   techniques, 114–15
shock, 226
simple suture, 118–21, 226
skin, 226
skin graft knives, 49
   Silver knife, 50
   Watson modification of the Humby Knife, 50
skin grafting, 16, 18, 28, 50
skin preparation solutions, 113–14
   alcoholic iodine solution, 114
   aqueous chlorhexidine, 114
   chlorhexidine in alcohol, 114
   chlorhexidine and cetrimide, 114
   povidone-iodine solution, 114
skin stapling, 169
skull fracture, 8
slings, vascular, 156, 157
spinal column
   hyperextension, 9, 11
   hyperflexion, 9, 11
splitting dissection technique, 161–2
steam sterilisation, 204, 205–6, 208
sterile field, 227
sterile technique, 187
   breaches, 217
   clean air, 190
   clean environment, 187–8, 189–91
   clean equipment, 191
   clean hands, 191
   clean staff, 189
   draping, 193–4
   gowning/gloving, 197–201
   no-touch technique, 203–4
   operative site disinfection, 188, 191–3
   principles, 187–8
   procedural site isolation, 188, 193–204
   skin preparation, 192, 194
      solutions, 192–3, 195
   sterilisation of tools, 188, 204–7
   surgical scrub, 191
sterilisation, 204
   chemical methods, 204–5, 206
      ethylene oxide, 204–5, 206–7, 209
      glutaraldehyde, 206, 207, 209
      hydrogen peroxide plasma, 206, 207, 209
   dry heat, 204, 206, 209
   ionising radiation, 205
   steam, 204, 205–6
      autoclave, 205–6, 208
      flash unit, 206, 208
      vacuum, 206, 208
sterility, 113, 217, 226
suckers, 83

American pattern (ENT), 84
Poole, 85
simple, 84
Simpson-Smith, 85
sump, 84–5
Yankauer, 84, 85, 169
surgical skills, 31, 112, 144
   attitude, 112
   debridement, 149–53
   dissection, 158–63
   excisions, 144–9
   haemostasis, 153–8
   incisions, 112, 114, 144–9
   instrument safety, 114–15
   positioning, of surgeon, 113
   sharps techniques, 114–15
   tissue blood supply, 115–16
   wound tension, 116
suture materials, 40, 91, 98–102, 108–9
   absorbable, 99, 101
      catgut, 100, 102–4, 118
      poliglecaprone 25, 106
      polydioxanone, 101, 105
      polyglactin, 910, 104–5
      polyglycolic acid (PGA), 104
      trimethylene/glycolic acid, 105
   absorption, 98, 99
   braided, 103
   choice of, 38
   monofilament, 98–100, 101, 103
   multifilament, 98–100
   natural, 102–4, 110
   nonabsorbable, 99, 101
      cotton, 101, 110
      linen, 101, 110
      polyamides, 107
      polybutester, 106
      polyester, 107, 110
      polyether, 106–7
      polypropylene, 107
      polyvinylidene, 106
      silk, 30, 99, 100, 101, 110
      stainless steel, 101, 110
   origin, 98, 99
   sizes, 102
   synthetic, 101, 104–7, 118
sutures, 28, 30
   cutting, 168–9
   defined, 227
   following, 167–8
   size, 91, 97–8
suturing techniques, 91, 116–17
   Barron suture, 126, 129
   continuous suture, 125
   horizontal mattress suture, 124–5
   placement of sutures, 117
   principles, 117–18
   simple suture, 118–21
      buried, 119
      everting, 119
      inverting, 119
   subcuticular suture, 126, 127–8
      bridge, 126, 128
   three-corner suture, 129
   vertical mattress suture, 122–3
swab-on-a-stick, 167, 169
swaging, 91, 92, 93, 95–7
synapse, 227

tension, 28, 116, 227
tetanus, 36

Index

theatre environment, 115
thermal energy injury, 6, 16
  cold, 12–13, 16, 18–19, 21, 22
  heat, 6, 12–13, 16–18
thoracic aorta, 9–10
threshold potential, 227
thrombocytopenic patients, 154
tissue forceps, 53–60
tissue planes, 223
tissues
  blood supply, 115–16
  displayed, 158–60
  distraction, 159
  excitable, 223
  exposure of, 223
  loss of, 1
topical anaesthesia, 181
tourniquets, 154, 156, 182, 216
  arterial, 154, 156
towel clips, 85–6
  ratcheted scissors-pattern, 86
  spring-action, 86
toxicity, defined, 227
trauma
  blunt, 6, 10, 12, 18
  penetrating, 6, 10, 12, 14–15, 18
trenchfoot, 16, 18, 22, 227
trimethylene/glycolic acid, 105

Universal Precautions, 214, 227
urinary catheterisation, 188

vascular clamps
  crushing (haemostatic), 60–1
  non-crushing, 60, 62, 65–6, 156
    Bulldog, 66
    Debakey angled, 65
    Satinsky, 66
vascular slings, 156, 157
vesicle formation, 21
vessels, 71
  clamps, 156
  control, 154–8
  ligation, 154, 155, 158
  oversewing, 154, 156, 158
  slings, 156, 157
  transfixion, 154, 156, 158

warfarin, 154
wound healing, 1, 24, 26
  delayed primary closure, 25, 38, 222
  first intention healing, 24–5, 27, 38, 223
  general factors affecting, 28, 30–1
  local factors, chronic tissue factors, 29–30
  local factors affecting, 28, 30
    contamination, 29
    dead space, 29, 118
    foreign bodies, 29
    haematoma, 29
    irradiation, 30
    ischaemia, 28
    local trauma, 29
  sutures, 30
  wound infection, 29
  wound tension, 28
  second intention healing, 25, 26–7, 226
  technical factors affecting, 28, 31
wound management, 1, 32, 39
  antibiotics, 35–6
  assessment
    criteria for seeking expert help, 35
    need for closure, 33, 35
    wound mechanism, 6–24
    wound type, 1–5
  decision-making schema, 34
  evaluation, 31, 32–3
  examination, 33
  explanation to patient, 35
  history, 32
  informed consent, 35
  method of repair, 33
wound mechanism, 6
  chemical injury, 6, 13, 21, 23
  electrical injury, 6, 13, 23
  ionising radiation injury, 6, 13
  kinetic energy (blunt) injury, 6–10, 12
  kinetic energy (penetrating) injury, 6, 10, 12, 14–15
  thermal energy (cold) injury, 6, 12–13, 18–19, 21, 22
  thermal energy (heat) injury, 6, 12–13, 16–18
wound repair, 33
  anaesthesia, 36
  antimicrobials, 35–6
  choice of suture material, 38
  closure, 38, 169
  debridement, 37
  dressings/splints, 38
  haemostasis, 37, 153–8, 169
  post-repair, 38–9
  pre-repair, 33–6
  sterile field, 37
  wound preparation, 36–7
wounds
  causes, 6, 12–13
  classification, 4–5
  dead space, 29, 118
  high-velocity
    penetrating, 10
    projectile, 15
  incised, 224
  increase in strength over time, 27
  infection, 2, 18, 29, 118
  low-velocity, penetrating, 10, 14
  reclassification, 2
  site, 1
  tension, 28, 116, 227
  type 1, 2, 3, 4
  type 2, 2, 3, 4
  type 3, 2, 3, 4
  type 4, 2, 3, 5

xylocaine, 36